My Life's Lemonade

Lemonade

The Bitter and the Sweet

But there is a spirit in man: and the inspiration of the Almighty giveth them understanding. The spirit of God hath made me, and the breath of the Almighty hath given me life.

Job 32:8, 33:4

Jo Ann Speer Martin

MISSION POSSIBLE PRESS, USA
Creating Legacies through Absolute Good Works
Extraordinary Living Series

The Mission is Possible.
Sharing love and wisdom for the young and "the young at heart," expanding minds, restoring kindness through good thoughts, feelings, and attitudes is our intent. May you thrive and be good in all you are and all you do…
Be Cause U.R. Absolute Good!

My Life's Lemonade, *The Bitter and the Sweet*
Copyright © 2014 Jo Ann Speer Martin

Published by
Mission Possible Press
A Division of Absolute Good
P.O. Box 8039, St. Louis, MO 63156
Email: orders@absolutegood.com

ISBN 978-0-9852760-7-2

Dedication

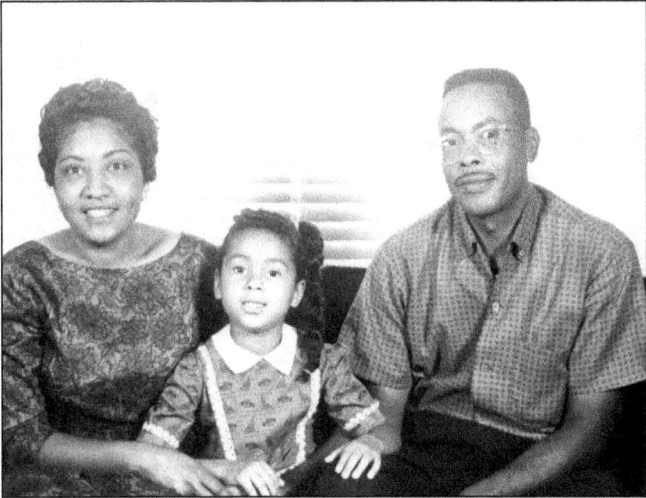

Mom, Dad and Jo Ann at 6 years old

To James and Helyn Speer, my parents. You wanted a child and could not have one so you adopted me and raised me as your own in a God-fearing home with a strong religious foundation. Our home was full of love and I am grateful you picked me for your very own. I carry you in my heart daily.

To "My Boo," Marty (Garnel Martin), the love of my life. You are my best friend, my provider, my lover, and you have continued to be my stabilizer. Thank you for pampering me throughout our marriage and for continuing to nurse me, especially during the writing of this book. You complete me.

I also dedicate this book to the many people who have been placed in my life by God for a reason during various seasons of my life. For fear that I will forget someone extremely important

I won't call names. But to my spiritual leaders, all of my family, my closest friends, my bosses, my social organization sisters and brothers, you have all had a great hand in who I have become. Thank you.

Without encouragement and faith in God I would not have been able to overcome the obstacles that life brought me. To God be all the glory.

Contents

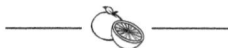

I Am Blessed

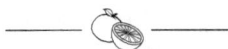

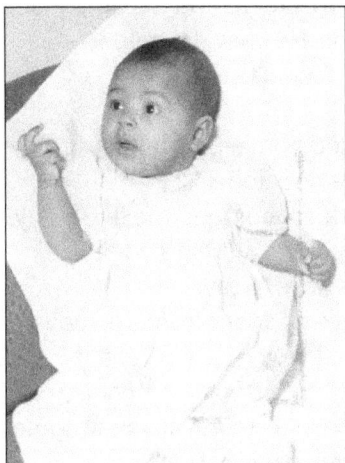

Jo Ann at 4 months old

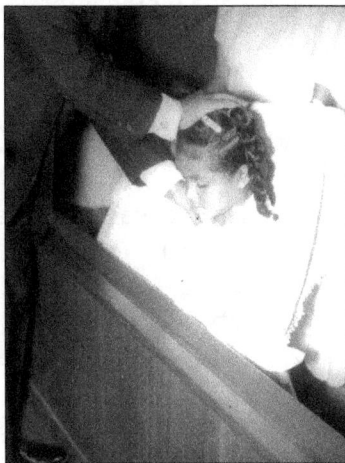

Jo Ann Baptism 1964

Oh what a blessed life I live.
Yes I've had my share of ups and downs.
What helped through them all is who I found.
From day one a special child I have been
Everyone told me but I didn't know then.

From before you were born He knew the hour and time of day.
He knew *me* by name and in which family I would stay.
If I had to choose my parents I'd do it the exact same way.
It's their love and teachings that made me who I am today.

I was special so He placed me in the best of them all.
They were the ones to raise me and teach me to stand tall.
The foundation was laid to keep Him with me at all times.
I am never alone for my joy in Him I find.

From a very early age Jesus was my friend, but as
I got older I really let Him in.
I know He always has my back and there's really
nothing that I lack.
There was a moment though I lost focus and became mad.
But Jesus never left me, He knew I would
be back when I wasn't sad.

When my parents were called home, God made sure
on earth I was not alone.
My family that was left on earth encouraged me every day.
I am still surrounded by love and that's what
all my families have to say.
My husband, I am very positive was sent from up above.
After 27 years we are still very much in love.

My life is great and always has been. Through all my struggles
God holds my hand.
I didn't always feel it when I was going through,
But I was taught He is forever faithful and this I always knew.

Sometimes we need proof to know that God has never left us.
He does just what He promised even when we raise a fuss.
I am so glad that I found Him, He has blessed me since birth.
He remains the head of my life, and I hope I live what He thinks
I'm worth.

Jo Ann Speer Martin

Getting Started

I don't even really know where to start. I want this to be an inspirational book. For more than twenty years I have heard my friends and family say I should write a book. I admit, my life has been pretty unique. Being an adopted German child, having retired as a Lieutenant Colonel from the Air Force, and having lived through over 20 surgical procedures does make me a candidate for a compelling life story.

I really like writing poetry, but I never even seriously thought about writing a book on any topic. So many people have told me, "Just put your thoughts on paper, put a cover on it and sell it." But I have always thought of writing a book to be a lot more than that. I had to think of grammar, spelling, the order, if pictures should be included or not, proofing, context and so much more. There were so many things to consider. Oh, when I started to get this book all in order, I wish I had listened to my friends years ago and started saving events in my life. Yet, as I started writing I realized it was so much bigger than punctuation or pictures.

Living or Dying

The past three years caused me to say to myself, *Jo Ann you should write a book!* Yes, I am brave and strong; yet, I started writing and would not stop until I told my story because this time, I thought I would die. It's not pretty, it's not easy to say, but it is true. My body has been through so much. Though my mind has been made up, I just didn't know if my body would cooperate and heal again.

Being diagnosed with Breast Cancer after the many other illnesses was kind of my last straw. I am an optimistic helpful person who enjoys being active. I am also human. I was tired. When I think about the people I have met along the way, they have helped me make it through. Some days I got up for my husband more so for myself. Some of the people I met in the hospitals and their families, I can honestly say, encouraged me with my own story at critical times when I was just tired. I choose to live.

I must admit I took on this project, "writing a book," like it was one of my major endeavors in the military, it's my story after all. You don't just become Lieutenant Colonel in the Air Force without earning it, especially when you look like me. I had to earn it. Being a leader and being in charge or at least "in control" is natural for me. I like it, I'm a natural, and I take care of my people. So I started getting things lined up, researching, connecting, putting my thoughts in the computer. I was driven to tell what was appropriate and to honor those who have been so good to me. I also needed dates and facts and such. That's efficient and necessary. Sounds good, right?

One day I realized I had gathered materials, written sentences, crafted paragraphs and "done my part." I was satisfied. The facts, events and pictures were all lined up, in order and ready for editing and publication. My book was finished but my life is not.

Reaching Out

No matter what happens in life, if you don't give up, you can make it. And even when you want to give up, you can still make it. It may not be easy, but you can make it. I don't think all obstacles can be conquered alone. Sometimes you have to ask for help to conquer obstacles. I know a lot of people let pride get in the way and they won't ask for help. You may be missing a blessing if you don't reach out.

I've been sick a lot and my husband asks me every time I get sick why I put it on the internet and on FB. He says, "Why do you tell everybody everything?" I tell him that I don't tell everything but, if I share what's happening with me and I ask for people to pray for me, I need to be specific so that they'll know what to pray for. Because there is power in prayer and I can feel the results of those prayers.

Emotionally things don't necessarily seem easier but things seem to be easier to accept when I know that others are also praying for my health and for the same thing I am praying for. I have so many people that have said to me, "Oh my goodness, you're a strong woman." I tell them that I'm strong from my faith in God and the strength I pull from those that love me. I have received well, over 1,000 emails and FB messages encouraging me, acknowledging they are praying for me, and they are inspired by my strength in the last year alone.

It feels good to recall how others have found strength and courage during my times of struggle and challenges. Now it's time to give until I have nothing left. I can't control my body but I choose to live. I can't force myself to have energy but I can be gentle with myself and rejuvenate. I don't like to talk about certain feelings but I do have them and willingly share them when I see a person needs encouragement. I don't want to tell you I have been scared but I won't lie and say I have not.

Perhaps you will find some inspiration, delight or just insights which will make your life better through hearing about some of my experiences. I am just happy to be right here, having listened to my friends and to my own heart, telling my story, and maybe encouraging you along the way.

What Can You Learn From My Life?

You can't have sweet lemonade without a few bitter lemons. You can't overcome obstacles alone – you need earthly friends or family – a support system. God can do anything but fail; He says ask in His Word and receive. And though it may not be when I want it, or even what I asked for, I have learned that He knows what's best.

Make the best of your life. You may have one body however there is a power greater than you and me who is ultimately in control, in charge, the boss, the head honcho. When you are strong-willed, independent and efficient like me, it's hard to submit yet, who else could I trust my life or yours to? We have what we have. My faith makes me whole.

- Jo Ann Speer Martin

I'm a gentle strong spirit. I know how to stand up and I know how to back down. Most of my life I have put others before me. I have cussed people out and gotten into a few fights yet, most of my life, I have put others before me. I carry a large spot in my heart for the elderly and I love my family and God with all my heart.

We make or break our lives based on decisions and attitudes. We live or die based on faith, not based on diagnosis. We are born to people who may or may not parent us. We marry or we don't. We work hard or we become lazy. We appreciate people or we become bitter. We respect ourselves or we end up where we don't want to be. We inspire others when we do the best we can with what we've got, only if they want to be inspired. We keep secrets and sometimes that's good, sometimes it's not. We share our truth, or leave in mystery.

Live your life. Don't wait until it's too late. This is what I've got. I hope you enjoy it. It's still what I've got. Make the best of your life. If you don't like some of the lemons in your life, what make some sweet lemonade. You are still here so, I know you can do it. I've never really taken the obstacles that came to me in life as "challenges." I never really looked at them that way. I have just taken the life I was given and made the best of it.

I Am Still Here

I don't know the whole reason I'm still here but I sure hope I'm worthy. God has chosen for me to be here. I'm not sure I know what I've done to deserve that, but I am now more focused on living my life in a way that I would be worthy of living the life He has given me and that has not always been my focus.

Giving Thanks

—⟨🍊⟩—

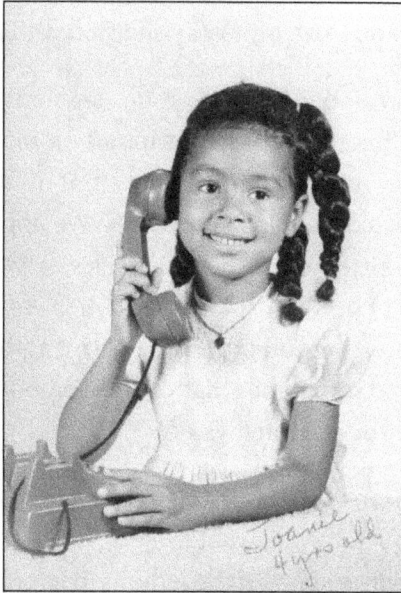

Jo Ann at 5 years old

Never Give Up

If you are ever down and out, you may always turn to the Lord. When you are down unless you already know about his goodness, you may not want to hear this yet, even those that know the Lord need earthly encouragement sometimes. While I was squeezing the lemons in my life I had encouragement. If someone said something to me which did not seem to be encouraging, I ignored it and 10 encouraging statements would follow. Believe me, during the last three years, I have

- Jo Ann Speer Martin

had some very down days. There were days when I did not want to try and get out of bed. Yet, I never stopped praying. I did all I could to get up spiritually, especially since my body wasn't always cooperating.

Give Thanks

Be thankful for the things you wouldn't give up anyway. It's real easy to tell somebody when they are down and out, "Don't give up, hang in there." But, we don't always tell people when they are sitting on the mountain top, enjoying everything about their life, they need to give thanks.

God is a selfish God. He wants us to praise Him for who He is and to be still and know that He is God. We don't always do that. He doesn't ask very much from us. We can ask, "God, please forgive me!" and in the snap of a finger, everything you have done is forgiven. He sacrificed His only son for our salvation. Some of us don't know that and some of us forget that. He deserves thanks.

Jesus and Me

———— 🍊 ————

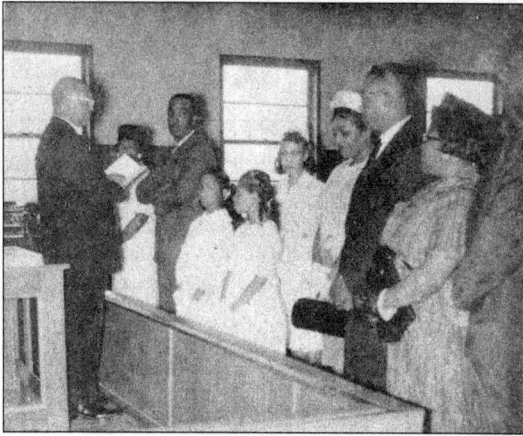

My First Baptism

I found out I was adopted at the age of seven from a friend at school who heard her mother talking about my situation. When I got home from school, I told my mother what she said. That night my parents sat me down and explained adoption to me in a way that I would understand. My mom said out of all the children in the world, she chose to have me as her very own and that *I was special* and I always would be special. They also told me not to listen to others because she and dad were my parents and nothing would ever change that.

I appreciate the way my parents handled the adoption conversation. They assured me I was loved, I was chosen, I was special and I was theirs. That's a powerful message for a seven year old and actually, for any person.

- Jo Ann Speer Martin

I have loved Jesus since I was a kid. When I was ten years old, I told my mom I wanted to join the church and be baptized. I had always been told God loved me so much that He let His son die so I may live and if I did what the Bible said, I would get to meet Jesus one day. I did not realize until I got older and was having some life experiences of my own, the impact of those words and how a few drops of water would change my life forever. I want people who love the Lord to think more about how God has affected their lives and the blessings they have received over the years. I want people to live with hope and to be inspired enough to help others be inspired.

The Power of Identity

If you have been adopted or have a child who is adopted, as adults, you have a responsibility to yourself and to your loved ones to make the very best out of the situation. Too often the subject of adoption becomes negative or painful, causing resentment or worse not necessarily because of the act itself, but because the way people handle it. If adoption has affected someone you or someone you love, remember truthfulness, sincerity and love are keys to identity, self-esteem and trust. No matter your age or situation, you can look at the past yet choose your future.

I'm a strong Black woman. My strength comes from God. He makes strength possible through my direct relationship with him, and also with my family and friends. They are all my support system. I know that He is with me. I feel it every day. He has proven that to me through events that have happened and continue to happen in my life. Ultimately, everything I am and have ever been is through Him. I am grateful.

My Parents, The Speers

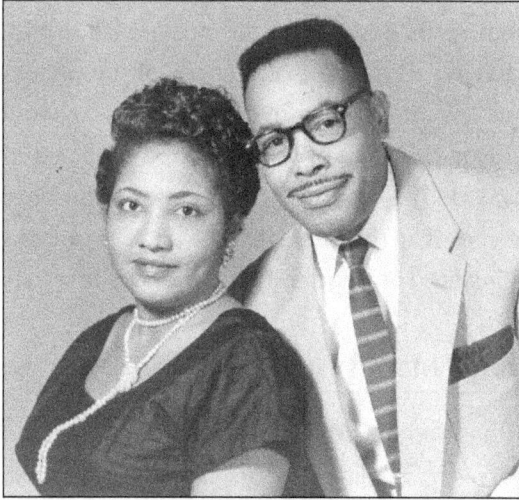

My Parents Back in the Day Helyn and James Speer

The family which adopted me, James and Helyn Speer, were the best parents in the world. I know everyone thinks they have the best parents, but mine were as special as they told me I was. My dad who, everyone called "Chick," was in the United States Army for 22 years. When he retired, he was hired as the Manager of University Stores at Grambling State University in Louisiana. I remember my mom having two different jobs when I was growing up. The first one was for the Social Security Office in Monroe, LA, which was a 60 mile commute every day. Eventually she started working at Grambling State University as the secretary for the Adult Education Office.

Family and Fun

There was never a dull moment in our house. As the only child, I remember taking vacations every year to Six Flags Over Texas in Arlington or to Six Flags AstroWorld in Houston. At first mom and dad would alternate who rode the scary rides with me, but it wasn't long before mom would bow out and let dad ride all the scary rides with me.

In the summers, I would go and stay at my mother's parents' house in Tallulah, Louisiana. Mylas and Mattie Baity were my grandparents, and they too were the best. I called them Grandma and Paw. Tallulah was only 90 miles from my house, so it was easy for me to see them often.

We also visited my dad's parents, Joseph (Daddy Speer) and Fay (Momma Fay) Speer in McDonough, Georgia. Before dad went to Korea, we were stationed at Fort Benning, Georgia, so I got to see them more when I was really young because we lived so close. I had so many cousins there. It was always fun visiting with them. Momma Fay was actually my dad's step mom; his mother died before I could meet her. My dad's family owned a funeral home and they still do, (Speer and Speer Funeral Home). I can remember playing in the funeral home as a child. Dad had two brothers and two sisters, William, Joseph, Fleta Mae and Josephine. I never met my Aunt Fleta Mae because she died at a young age. Her daughter, Barbara, runs the funeral home today. My Aunt Josephine is the only sibling who is still alive. She lives in Charlotte, North Carolina. We talk often and she calls me to pray.

Activities

My young years were great years. Mom and dad were always coming to see me performing or participating in various programs. I was involved in a lot of activities like dance, piano lessons and recitals, I played sports and I played in the band. I wasn't an angel though I was usually pretty good. Any one of my parents' friends had permission to spank me if they thought I was out of line and before I could get home they would have called to tell what I was doing.

Biking

My dad taught me how to ride a bike. Riding was fun back then. I don't know about now because it has been so long since I have been on a bike. I was told not to go out of the neighborhood. Well, to me that meant *if you go out of the neighborhood don't get caught.* I went riding down this big hill that was truly out of the neighborhood and wouldn't you know I fell? I skidded down the hill on my hip bone and leg as I dragged the bike with me. When I got to the bottom of the hill and saw all the blood, I panicked. I ran half way back up the hill to a friend of my parents' house and asked for help. Mrs. Henry met me at the door, saw all the blood, and panicked too. She told me to come in and laid me on her couch. She went to the bathroom to get some towels and try to clean me up. When she said I am going to call your Mom, I hollered, "No, you can't tell my mom." She didn't hear a word I said and called anyway. Oh my mom was so mad when she came to pick me up, I knew when I got home

- Jo Ann Speer Martin

I was going to "get it." I missed a spanking that time because mom and dad had to take me to the doctor.

Fishing

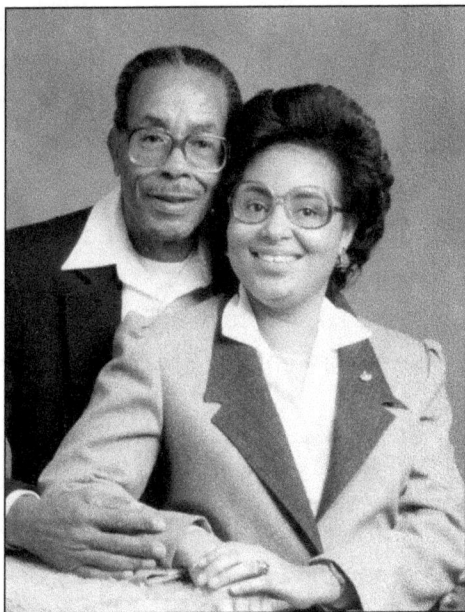

Dad & Jo Ann

I remember dad teaching me how to fish. Dad took me fishing in a boat even though mom had said, "I don't want you putting my baby in a boat." She was scared of boats because she didn't know how to swim. Since she didn't go with us that day, daddy put me in a boat anyway. While we were in the boat, a snake fell out of a tree into the boat. Daddy took the oar and was trying to beat the snake and the boat turned over. Now, I knew how to swim and daddy did too. But, the snake was in between me and Daddy and the snake was just skimming across the top of the water. Daddy grabbed the oar and was trying to beat at the snake and get to me, which he finally did. When we got out of the water and got the boat out of the water, Daddy said, "JoAnn, you can't tell you momma that you fell out the boat because she'll never let you go fishing with me again." And I replied, "Okay Daddy, I ain't going to tell her." We got home, walked in the door and momma said, "What are you doing so wet?" The first thing I said was, "Momma, the boat turned over in the water and there was a snake in the boat." Oh! My Daddy got so mad! He said, "I told you not to tell her." I said, "Daddy, I had to tell her, she wanted to know why I was so wet." It was so funny, at least it was funny afterward. I did get to go fishing with Daddy again… however, whenever we went, momma had to go with us! And she always did.

Curiosity and Cussing

I had braids long enough for me to sit on. My Grandma had a ringer washer machine and of course, I had to try it out. I stuck a braid in the ringer and it sucked my hair right up to my ear so fast. I was screaming for help until my Grandma came and turned it off. I didn't know it had a backup button. She just backed my hair right out but I was still in trouble.

I also remember my mom telling the story of how I stopped cursing. My dad was an Army man and he could really curse. I picked up all his bad habits at a young age. I was about seven or eight one summer while staying with my Grandma and Paw

- Jo Ann Speer Martin

when I got caught "cussing" by Grandma. Grandma told me that Jesus would not love me if I said bad words and I must not say them again. That was it, I quit. When mom and dad came to pick me up, mom asked what Grandma did to stop me from using bad words. She had done everything; spanked me, punished me, washed my mouth out and nothing worked. When Grandma told her what happened mom said she was ready to spank me again because that was too easy!

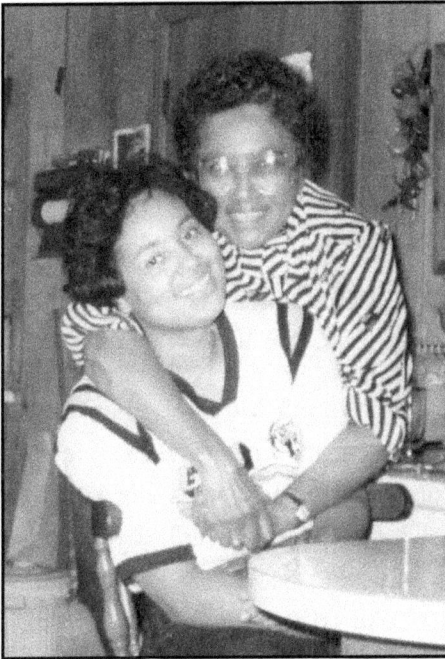

Mom and I in the Kitchen

Drinking

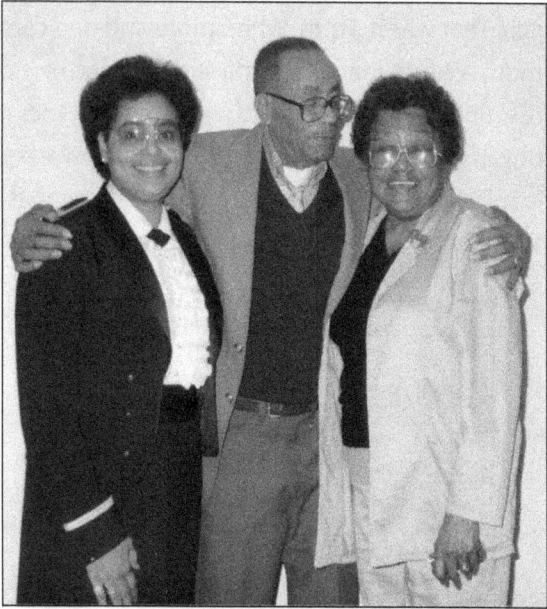

Dad, Mom and Me

Our family went through a lot together, as I am sure most families do. I remember while I was in high school my dad started drinking a lot and became an alcoholic. Our household was in turmoil for a while. One night while dad was out, mom woke me up and said, "Get dressed we are leaving." I was old enough to understand what was going on but I was kind of scared too. We left that night and moved into a hotel for about a week. Then some of my parent's friends came and we went and picked up all of our clothes, some furniture and kitchen stuff, and moved into an apartment. Dad knew what we were doing by then, and did not come home until we were finished. That

- Jo Ann Speer Martin

started a nine-year separation for my parents. They never got a divorce or legal separation, but we lived in separate homes. I was always back and forth because I wanted dad to know I still loved him. I did not spend the night with him though. I worked on getting dad sober for years and worked on mom forgiving him just as hard. When I would come home on military leave, I would have dad over to mom's house for dinner and they would get along fine.

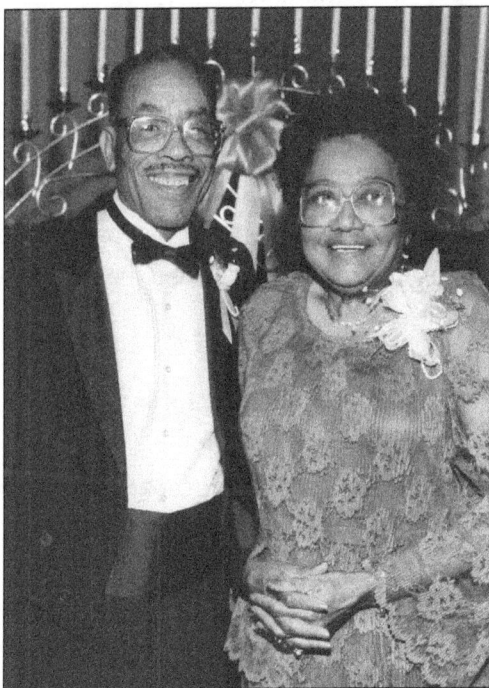

Mom and Dad on My Wedding Day

Everyone in Grambling knew my dad drank and drank all the time, so it was nothing I could hide. Mom's bout of alcoholism was covered up and kept secret, until now, except for the closest friends. It didn't last, but maybe a year. I remember it vividly because I couldn't figure out why she would do such a thing after living with an alcoholic for years. Mom's drinking was during my junior year in college and it made it rough on me trying to cover up another family secret. I didn't really have friends over when dad was drinking and now I couldn't have friends over because mom was secretly drinking. It was just more lemons for the lemonade.

Nine years after they separated mom called me and said they were getting back together, and she was moving back in the house. I was ecstatic, but couldn't really show it because I wanted it to be her decision. After all, I did not live there anymore. It really made me happy to know my parents were back in the same house. You know you can't have sweet lemonade without having some bitter lemons also.

Called Home

My father died in 1991 of bone Cancer and my mom in 1993 of diabetes. If dad had lived 2 more months they would have been married 50 years.

- Jo Ann Speer Martin

My Love, Marty

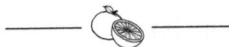

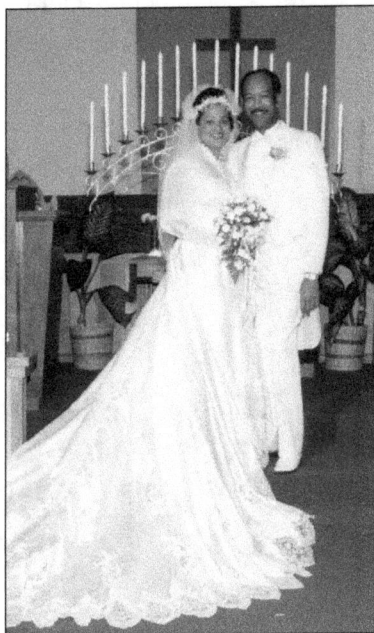

Our Wedding Day Mr. and Mrs. Martin

In 1986, I married Garnel Martin (Marty), who is 18 years older than me. My parents thought I was crazy at first. When they finally got to meet him they blessed our marriage. Marty retired after 23 years in the Air Force in 1978. He then worked 29 more years for McDonnell Douglas Aircraft and Boeing Aircraft. This man not only loves me but pampers me. He commuted as much as I did, if not more when we first got married and were living in separate places. Our marriage lasted for six years with us living in separate states. We never had time to get angry in the early years of our marriage because we were not together long enough to spend that time angry. If we did argue it wasn't long. What's great about it is we moved on, and the best thing is we are moving in the same direction. Our biggest argument now is where we are going to eat.

Meeting His Parents

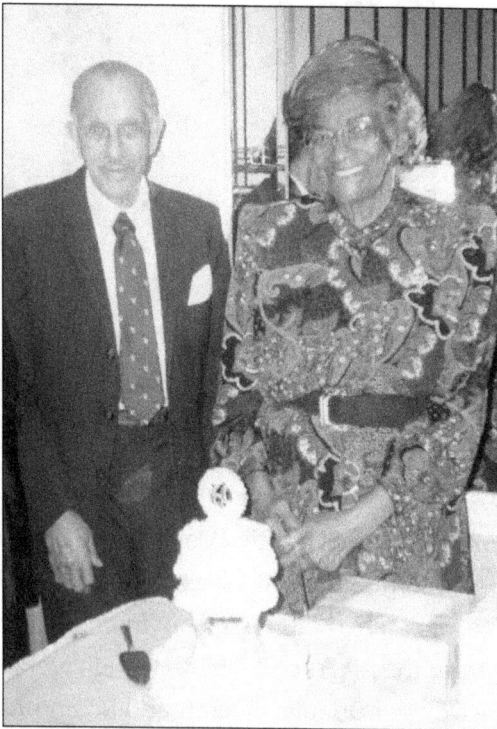

Daddy Carlisle & Momma Nellie 50th Wedding Anniversary

Before we were married, my parents made me explain to him about my birth and the fact that I could have blonde, blue-eyed children and they would still be his. He laughed and understood what I was saying. He took me to meet his parents before we married. You talk about being nervous? I was nervous. He told me as we drove to Virginia that his mother did not like for anyone to leave the walls in the bathroom wet when you finished showering. Do you know how the walls sweat after a good hot shower? Well, the first night I was in the bathroom forever trying to keep the walls dry. As fast as I dried them, they would steam right back up.

When I finally got out of the bathroom his mother asked, "What took you so long in there?" I replied, "I was drying the walls." She busted into laughter and said, "Why?" I told her what Marty had told me on the way there and she said, "Baby you can't believe everything he says!" We laughed about that for years.

Momma Nellie, as I fondly called her, was a gentle spirit. She read the Bible every morning and every night. She actually started me to reading the Bible because I had to read it to her. She and Daddy Carlisle, Marty's dad, were the center of the family. You know how you have one couple that everyone in the family goes to with everything? They were the ones. They accepted me into their family without question. Momma Nellie would tell people, "This is my daughter-in-law, but I leave the in-law off." Daddy Carlisle would sit and talk to me about the old days for hours and Marty couldn't understand why he wouldn't talk very much to anyone else. He was in general a very quiet man. Marty's cousins have treated me like a sister ever since I met them. They are all very close and include me in their circle. Everyone cannot say the same about their in-laws. Mine were great.

We lost Daddy Carlisle in 2002 to Alzheimer's at the age of 95. Momma Nellie was 96 when she passed in 2011 of heart failure. She too had Alzheimer's, but she always knew us when we visited.

Marty's Children

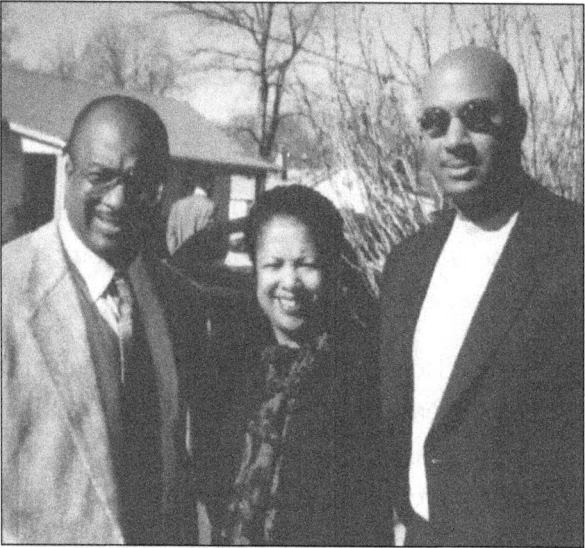

Garnel, Lyvia and Lionel

When Marty and I married, he had three kids from a previous marriage. They were already grown and living on their own when we got together. I was very nervous when we met because we were so close in age. I thought they would think I was a gold digger or something. That was not the case.

Garnel, Lydia, and Lionel accepted me as their dad's wife instantly. We have a wonderful relationship and talk to each other all the time. Lionel and Lydia came to Louisiana to our wedding. Garnel was working, so he could not make it but sent us best wishes. They got a chance to meet all of my family and we had a great time. They have been very supportive through my illnesses and call, checking on my progress often.

The love I knew growing up continues in this family because they make sure to show their love throughout the year and I do the same. It makes being a stepmother very easy when we all get along with love. I have heard "step mother stories" and did not want that to be the case in my life. I have great "step children" and their wonderful father as my best friend, provider and stabilizer to go right along with them. God once again blessed me.

Staying Married

Marriage is sacred and requires a lot of work. Open communication helps the relationship. It is OK to disagree. It doesn't mean divorce every time there is an argument. Hurry up and finish the argument so you can start to make up. Never go to bed without saying, "Good Night." Never get up in the morning without saying, "Good Morning."

PeeWee, My Biological Mother

———— ⊘ ————

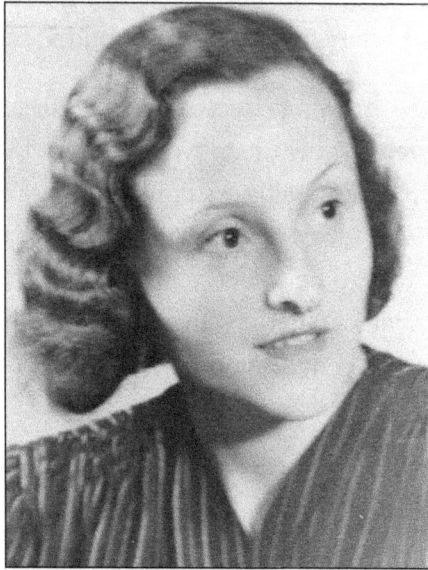

My Birth Mother PeeWee (Anna Reichman)

I was adopted in Germany at the age of 5 weeks by Black American Army parents. I was told by my parents at the age of seven that I was adopted. That is very young, but I understood what they said because they told me in a way I could understand.

As I got older I became more inquisitive about my birth parents. When I was a teenager my Mom gave me a picture she had received and been saving since my first birthday. It was a picture of a young white boy and a young Black girl. The boy looked around nine or ten and the girl around seven or eight

- Jo Ann Speer Martin

years old. My parents told me the pair was my brother and sister. Since both of my parents were Black, of course, I had many more questions! The biggest questions were, "Why?" and "How?" "What had I done at such an early age that would make my mother give me away?" And of course, "How could I have a brother that was white and a sister that was Black?"

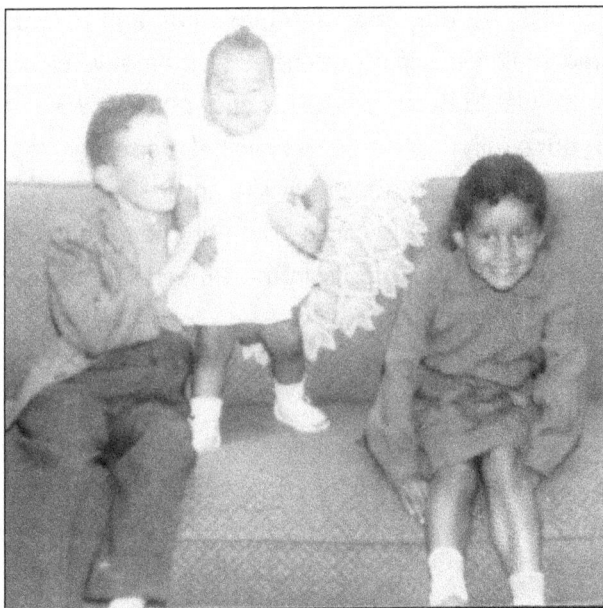

Peter, Me and Patricia - At Jo Ann's 1st Birthday in Her Parents Home

Learning About PeeWee and Me

PeeWee was a white German lady who had a boy with a white man. My sister and I had a Black father. As time passed my parents explained that my biological mother whom I refer to as "PeeWee," was not married when she gave birth to me, during a very poor time in Germany. PeeWee with three children already, thought it would be best for me if she gave me to a loving family who really wanted to raise and love a child as their own. They made it clear to me that her decision had nothing to do with what I had done or not done. These answers and explanations satisfied me for a while until I started to get sick quite often.

First tonsillitis all the time, then bronchitis, and my appendix ruptured while I was in high school. Each time we went to the doctor we would be asked the same questions, "Who has had this in your family?" "Did anyone have heart disease?" You know, relevant background questions like those. The answer was always, "I don't know," because I did not know. These illnesses stirred a continuous curiosity in me. I needed the answers to my medical background.

Searching for More

When I was in my late twenties, I started to contact embassies and adoption agencies in the US and in Germany to try and find details about my biological family. Fortunately, I had my adoption papers, which were written in both English and German, with some addresses from 1955 listed on them. With that, I began writing inquiries. This went on for many years. My parents were aware that I was looking for my biological mother and fortunately, they supported that effort.

In late 1982, my mom found in some of her old albums the address of a couple, Clifton and Erma Upton, who had been stationed in Germany with them. They were now living in

California. The couple knew I was adopted and also knew of one of PeeWee's friends. I reached out to them for information. Three months later the Uptons sent me the addresses for five of PeeWee's friends, including the address of Irmgard Murry, who still lived in Germany. I wrote each of them the same letter, explaining who I was and that I was looking for my biological mother, Anna Riechman (PeeWee). I wanted them to tell me what they knew even if it was, "She does not want to meet you." I then sat back and anxiously awaited an answer from all of them. Ms. Murry was the only one who wrote back. She told me that she did know PeeWee and that she did want to meet me. The letter provided me PeeWee's address and phone number. She had given PeeWee my address and phone number as well.

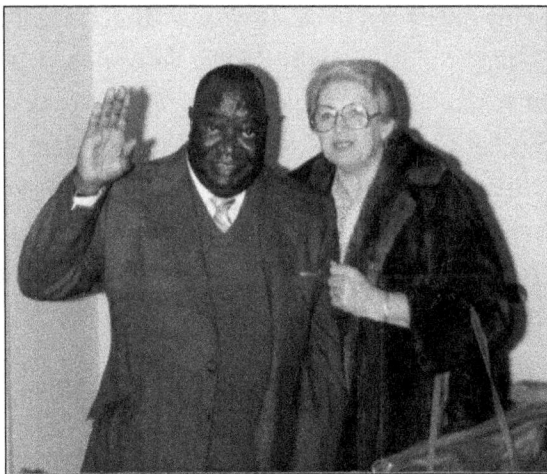

Clifton and Irma Upton, They Reconnected Our Family

I can still feel the excitement the day I received the letter. The people in my office kind of lived this part of my life with me because they all knew my story. They were all excited for me as well. At this time, I was in the United States Air Force and assigned to the Air Force Communications Command Inspector General Team at Scott Air Force Base, IL. This team traveled all over the country inspecting other bases. The day I received the letter, I went to the travel planners in our office and asked them to schedule me for any upcoming trip to Germany. I needed to be part of that team. I explained my situation and they said, "We will see." I couldn't wait to get off work to call my mom and tell her about the letter.

My parents and I were like peas in a pod; very, very close. Just before calling my mom, I thought what would be going through her mind after I told her. I have no doubt she knew she would be my 'only mom' because we were that close. But from a mother's stand point, I thought, *Would she wonder if I would love her less after finding my biological mother?* It had to take a lot for her to put her emotions aside and help me to find PeeWee. I was gentle when I called her but very honest. I was excited and my parents were excited also. I told them my concerns and they assured me if it had not been for PeeWee, they would not be my parents and they were happy for me.

In 1983, I was put on a team going to Germany for an inspection. A man named Tom Lacy was on our team. He was very familiar with Germany and spoke the language well. He told me if I wanted to take leave and stay a week after the inspection, he would borrow a friend's car. He was willing to drive me to meet PeeWee and stay until I was ready to come home, acting as a translator.

- Jo Ann Speer Martin

We made the trip and stayed a week.

When Tom and I found PeeWee's home, I was so nervous. We walked up to the door and I refused to knock. I told Tom I had changed my mind and wanted to leave. Tom took me to a pay phone so I could call my mom back in the states. I explained to her we found the house, but I had changed my mind and decided not to meet her. I said I would stand around the corner and just see her whenever she came outside.

My mom said to me; "I know you are nervous, but you have been searching a long time and if you give up now, you will never forgive yourself. Go back and knock on the door."

Tom told me the same thing, "You have come so far, don't give up now."

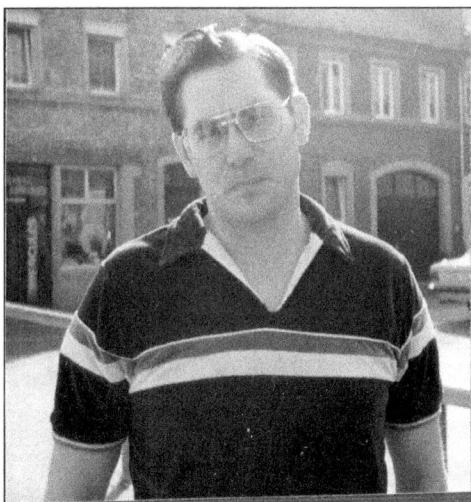

Tom Lacy

We went back. Tom knocked on the door and ran out of the way. PeeWee saw me out of her window and started calling me, "Jo Anna, Jo Anna!" She opened the door and gave me a big bear hug. She was a very small lady and came up to about my shoulder. I hugged her back, but I did not have all of the emotions that she had.

I think PeeWee was welcoming home a daughter that she had given a chance in life by giving her up. For me, I was meeting a total stranger that gave me away. I was not angry, but very curious and glad she still wanted to meet me after all these years. I had a million questions and some were answered and some were not. It was a very emotional time for both of us. Even in the middle of all of our excitement I thought about mom and dad back home and what were they thinking. We didn't have cell phones back then and I would not put a long distance call on PeeWee's phone bill, so I didn't talk to mom until I left PeeWee's house a week later.

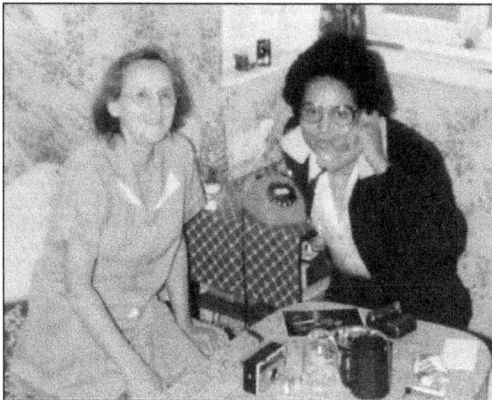

PeeWee and Jo Ann

When I talked with my parents, I let them know that my emotions were a lot different than I had expected them to be. Mom had never let me talk bad about PeeWee in any way. I had always known she had three children with three different fathers, but I did not know she had five children with five different fathers and I was the only one she gave away. PeeWee expressed some guilt for giving me away, but explained that it was a time of war and she could not handle another child right then. She wanted me to have a good life and so, she did what she thought was the best thing to do. She was really happy about the way I turned out.

While I was there, we went to the market every day and one night I took her out to dinner. We enjoyed our stay together and she really was happy to see me. She avoided the questions about my father and by the time I left, I had agreed that if she put me in touch with all of my siblings, I would not look for my father. She simply admitted he was Black, in the US Army and she said I she never told him she was pregnant. I have told myself that she probably did not tell him she was pregnant because he was married. I'll never know.

When I left Germany, I had my work cut out for me to contact my siblings and process mentally what I had just gone through. Both PeeWee and I were very happy about the meeting and vowed to keep in touch, which we did.

If you were adopted don't dwell on why you given away. Think of the happiness and the opportunities that are afforded you with parents that love you. If you adopted a child let them know it was because you wanted someone to love and teach and that they were chosen.

PeeWee made her decisions. I am glad we had the time and space to connect and get to know each other. Certainly our visit did not make up for the years we were separated but, it didn't need to. I had my parents. Upon meeting her, I gained a biological mother and my siblings. It could have been bitter but we all handled it well. I am grateful for the sweet lemonade.

Meeting My Siblings

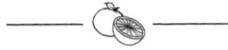

———— ✿ ————

When I left Germany I had phone numbers and addresses for all five of my siblings. I had actually talked to my baby sister, Peggy, who has lived in Germany all of her life, before I left the country. I was feeling very comfortable talking to her. She had a lot of questions and so did I.

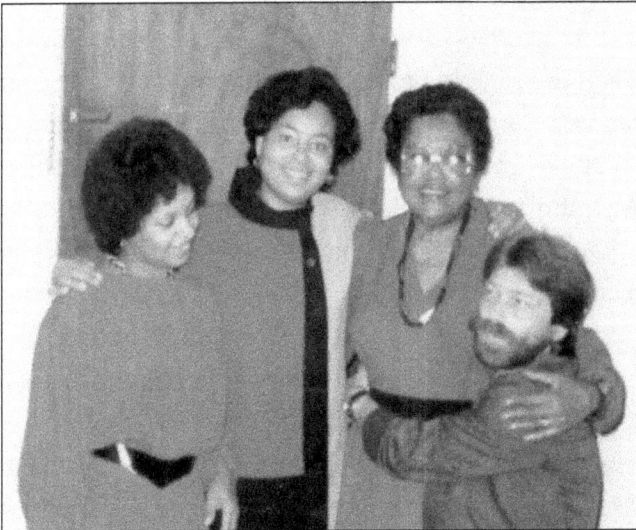

Peggy, Jo Ann, Mom and Elmar

Peggy And Elmar Visit Illinois

After returning to the states, I started saving money to bring Peggy and her fiancé, Elmar, over for a visit. We talked back and forth on the phone and a two-week trip was planned. At that time, I was still in the Air Force and living in O'Fallon, IL.

During the first week, Peggy and Elmar stayed at my house. It was just like catching up on old times. We were definitely sisters. We had so much in common. I showed them around the St. Louis area and we talked with my parents, who were living in Louisiana, almost every day. They really wanted to meet Peggy, so I decided to take her and Elmar to visit them that next week.

My parents were so excited that they were like children. They had a big reception at a Holiday Inn and invited about 150 people to meet Peggy and Elmar. They really hit it off with one of the guests, an old professor in college who taught German. It was very surprising to me how very well both Peggy and Elmar spoke English. We had no communication problems at all. My mom's sister, Aunt Flo and her husband, Uncle Al had a barbeque at the Mayor's house, who was very good friends with our family and lived across the street. I invited some of my friends to the barbeque and we all had a great time. I was in my world because everybody was getting along. I remember Peggy and I laying on my mother's bed and trying on all of her jewelry and hats just like little kids. We had a wonderful time in Louisiana. When the time came to put Peggy and Elmar on the plane, it was a tearful departure.

I had asked Peggy if she thought the other brother and sisters would like me. She assured me they would. I sat down and wrote my brother, Peter and his wife Rosie. They lived in Canada and still do. I told them all about me, the good and the bad. I

- Jo Ann Speer Martin

knew Peggy had already talked to them. Can you imagine after twenty some years a person comes up and says, "Hi I'm your sister?" I am sure it was a shock for their whole family.

Thanksgiving With Peter And Rosie

I talked with Peter and Rosie off and on and then I planned a trip to meet them. Peggy's father lived in Detroit, Michigan and Peggy was planning a trip to the states to have Thanksgiving with the family. The Thanksgiving celebration was in Detroit and Peter and his family would be there also. Peggy flew to Toronto to Peter's, and the whole family drove down to Detroit. I was on a trip with the Air Force in Hawaii and could not be there until two days after Thanksgiving. My new family postponed the Thanksgiving Dinner Celebration until I could get there. They were so thoughtful and sweet to do that just for me. I have tears in my eyes even as I write this.

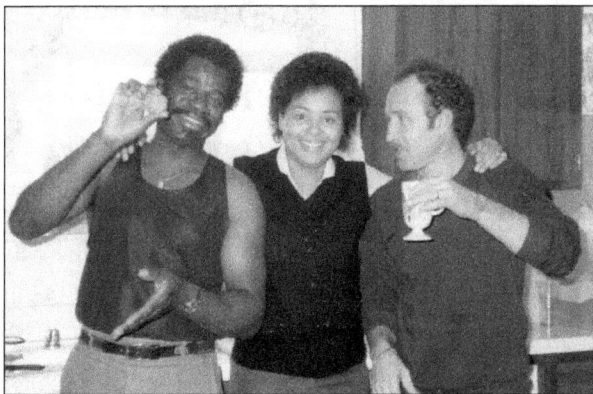

Thanksgiving Morning Peggy's Dad Melvin, Jo Ann and Peter

I arrived in Detroit and Peggy and Peter met me at the airport. My emotions and adrenaline were indescribable. It was really like a dream come true. We were there three days and it was a wonderful time. Being in the house with that many family members at one time after growing up an only child was so exciting for me. Peter had four kids; Monica, John, Anne and Petra. They were young at the time and I loved kids, so we played and horsed around together. It was just like we had grown up together.

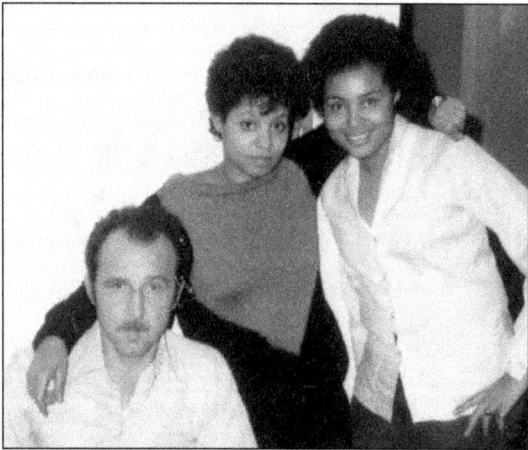

Siblings Peter, Peggy and Jo Ann Celebrating Thanksgiving

I can remember sitting on the couch, idly shaking my leg up and down like I frequently did. Rosie hit my leg. I asked her why she hit me. She said, "Your brother shakes his leg like that all the time and it makes the room vibrate." We both laughed and I said, "It runs in the family." Thinking of that really makes me smile as Peter and I looked quite a bit alike and we hit it off really great. There are so many things we have in common.

- Jo Ann Speer Martin

Most of the family says we both have German tempers. That tickles us both.

After that visit I tried to keep up with everyone's birthday and send presents or cards and we talked all the time. I just love it when the kids called me Aunt Jo Ann. They aren't kids anymore. They are adults with their own families but they still call me Aunt Jo Ann.

My Sister Karin

As I mentioned before, PeeWee gave birth to five children. Karin is the oldest sibling and Patricia is between Peter and me in age. For years most of us often kept in touch. I took a while however, 12 years after meeting PeeWee, I got to meet Karin and her family.

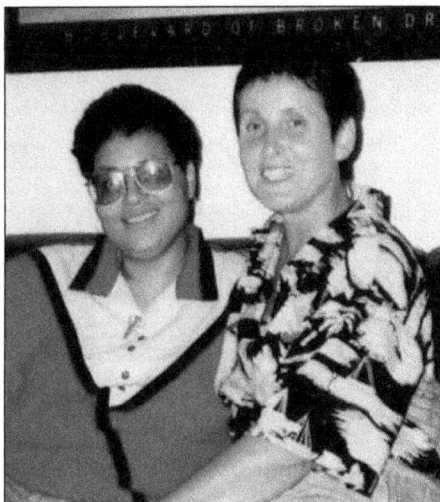

Sisters Jo Ann & Karin

In 1995, Peter threw a big birthday party in Canada and Karin and her husband, Hans Pape were flying in from Germany to attend the party. It was the perfect time for me to meet Karin. Karin does not speak a lot of English, but Peter and Peggy would be there to translate what we could not figure out. I spoke a little German back then, but it is gone now.

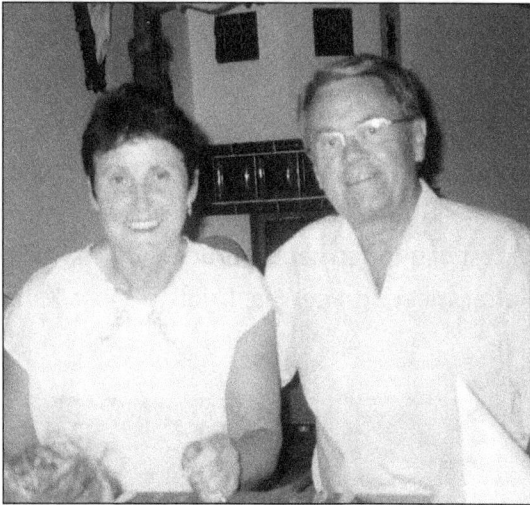

My Sister and Her Husband Karin and Hans Pape

Marty and I planned to be there. All of the emotions and excitement started up again for me. I couldn't wait to meet her. In spite of the language barrier, we got along very well. Karin and Hans have two daughters; Darja and Dorothee, who I haven't yet met. Dorothee has two sons; Hurbertus and Ludwig. All of them still live in Germany. I'm really glad we got that chance to spend time together as Hans passed in 1998. Karin and I are still in touch and my niece, Darja, translates for us. I have pictures of

- Jo Ann Speer Martin

all the family and they have pictures of our little family also. We also exchange gifts on birthdays and Christmas, but I don't get to talk to them much anymore. I really miss that.

My Sister Patricia

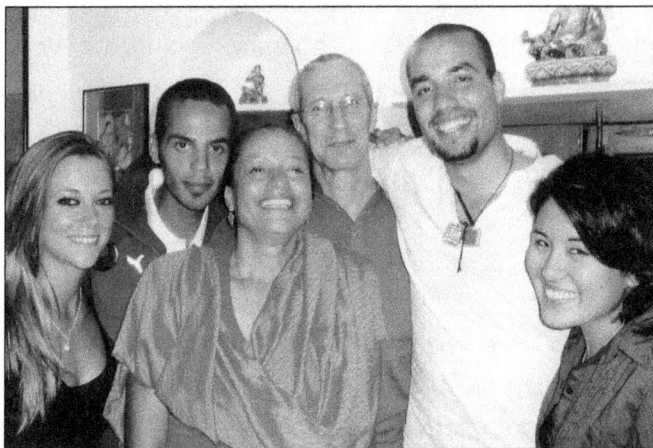

My Sister Patricia with Her Husband Phillipe Recent Family Photo

When I moved to Germany permanently for my Air Force assignment in 1985 I was in touch with PeeWee often. The month after I arrived, the Air Force was delivering my household goods and PeeWee called me. Guess who was in town visiting her mother? It was Patricia, who is right above me in age. She wanted me to come to Kitzingen, where she was, for a visit. She spoke English very well, but with an accent. I tried to explain to her that the Air Force movers were at my house unloading furniture and I could not leave that day. I could come the next day, but she was leaving the next day. I enjoyed talking to her, but it wasn't a long conversation and I have not heard from her since.

Patricia lives in Katmandu, Nepal with her husband Phillipe. They have two boys who are young men now; Raphael, and Sumpten. I have pictures of her and her family from various years. We really look alike. All of the other sisters and my brother keep me up to date on how she is doing, but even they don't get to talk or see her often. I do have meeting her and her family on my bucket list, along with all of us taking a family portrait together.

My Unique Family

I have never been a half way person so all of my sisters and my brother are never referred to as half brothers and sisters unless I am talking to a doctor. All of us that I have met have established a relationship as if we grew up together. Over the years, they have met my adoptive family and I have met all of their family members and life is good. When I retired from the Air Force, over 30 members of my families were present from all around the world. I can't tell you how that made me feel.

Family and Adoption

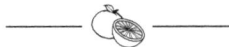

So many times the finding of biological parents does not work out like my story. In hindsight, I think God provided me a happy story with a new family that loves me and that I love because I was going to lose both my parents and He knew how important family was to me. Peggy is the only sibling who got a chance to meet my parents and she is also the only sibling whose father I have met. My siblings tell me I had the best of both worlds and I know this to be true. I have never referred to any of my family as "adoptive" or "biological"; nor would I typically refer to Marty's children as "step" but I separated them just for the purpose of this book. As my dad used to say, "Family is family."

I don't have a lot of comments for those who are adopting children other than, "Thank you." Make sure that child at some point knows that they were adopted. Pick their level of maturity to tell them and wait for them to ask questions. The questions will come in time. Let them know they are in your family because someone was willing to give up a child, for whatever reason, and that they were selected as their/your child.

Adoption is not temporary; it is a family heart string which cannot be broken. Make sure the child feels comfortable talking to you about their adoption and don't push them into knowing more than they want to know for that moment. Communication and the showing of love will do all the rest. Prepare them if they ever want to find biological family members, that the outcome may not be as positive as mine was but don't dwell on it.

Find Joy In Adoption

For those children who were adopted and know it, know that you were selected by the family that you call mom and dad. They could have selected anyone but they chose you. You will always have questions in your mind. Some will be answered during your life and some won't. Don't ever forget the value of family and those who love you. Don't miss a blessing in your current life worried about what might have been. Thank God for the love which surrounds you and if you find out more about your biological family consider it an added blessing. I call my family the rainbow family for the obvious reasons but the bottom line is there is no separation. We are all one big happy family.

My DNA

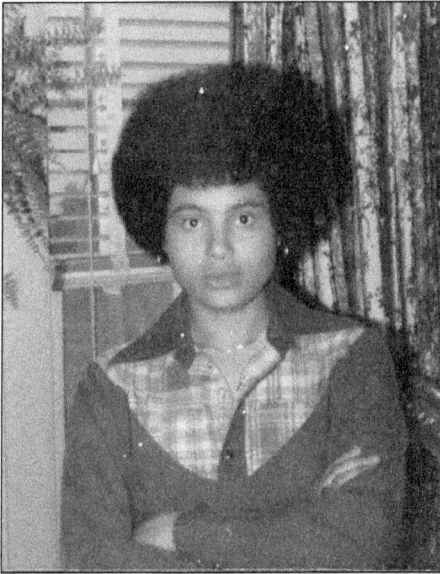

Me & My Afro

When I looked for my biological family, both of my parents were quite supportive however, my father was not real verbal. Now that they are both gone, my family members have urged me to look for my biological father. Most of them think my dad was my biological father. Though I have not yet shared about my biological mother whom I call PeeWee, I made a promise to her, upon our meeting. She asked me to promise not to search for my biological father if she put me in touch with my siblings. Her making that request, coupled with the fact that I look like all of my "adopted" cousins makes me say, "Hmmm." They all want me to do DNA testing, but in my heart, Daddy was the only daddy I will have.

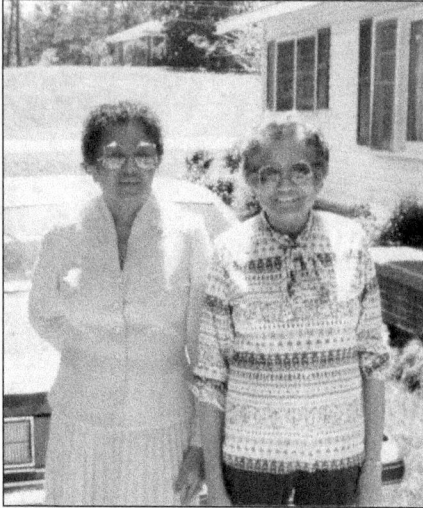

Mom and Her Sister Aunt Flo in the Yard

Some of my father's family just recently found out I was adopted. I just wonder why he didn't tell them, since he told everybody else. I also think about my Momma, Helyn. If, in fact, my Daddy was my daddy, she would have killed him for getting together with Pee Wee. Even though she is on the other side, I wouldn't want to think of her being hurt or upset, if she didn't know "the truth." I have decided not to do the testing. At this point, it wouldn't matter if I found another father, especially one that I didn't even know I existed, if that were the case. My dad (hero) and my mom (best friend), my parents remain.

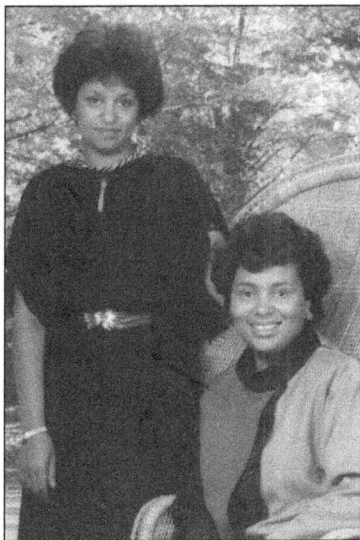

Peggy and Jo Ann

Being Family

Always remember *family* is one of the most important things in life. Stick together, play together, fight together and pray together. Family and friends are blessings from God and most of the time you get to pick who you want around you. Pick positive friends. Remember family is defined by heart strings not by bloodlines.

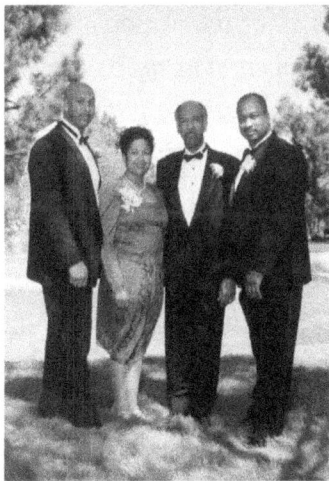

Lionel, Lyvia, Marty and Garnel

Bitterness and Restoration

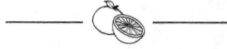

Family was important to me and it still is, but when I lost both of my parents, my world crumbled. I was raised in the church, but losing my parents made me turn away from the church. I loved my husband dearly but he couldn't replace my parents or the emptiness I felt with them gone. My self-esteem, my job and social life were affected.

In 2001, I had returned to the church and was singing in the choir. One day, I attended a workshop where we had to write a testimony and read it aloud. I will share that testimony with you.

Oh what an awesome God we serve! In the last 46 years that statement has taken on a new meaning for me each year. Each year I became a little closer, knew a little more, trusted a little further, and every year said, "This is the year that statement will mean the most to me." I grew up in a God-fearing family and with each new Christian friend I became closer to Christ. My Lord treated me special from birth. He placed me in a family that would provide me the Christian foundation I needed to grow into a Servant of the Lord. I was adopted at the age of 5 weeks old and my parents were and, although not here with me in physical form anymore, are still special. What I am about to tell you will explain what an understanding, forgiving, and delivering Father I have. Oh, my God is an AWESOME GOD. My faith was rock strong and steadfast until tragedy struck with a pain that stopped time for me.

- Jo Ann Speer Martin

In 1993 I, as an only child had lost both of my parents. My father died of Cancer in July 1991 and now my mother of diabetes in 1993. All of a sudden I could no longer hug my best friend or kiss my hero. My world began to quickly crumble. I lost my drive, my self-confidence, and my will. I became so angry with God that I had accepted as my Savior when I was seven years old that my world turned black and gloomy. (Psalms 34:18 - The Lord is close to the brokenhearted and saves those who are crushed in spirit.) I stopped sharing God's mercies with others, stopped going to church, stopped praying, and even cursed a God that would dare hurt me so bad and leave me so alone while surrounded by people.

I became very ill with many things happening at once; bleeding ulcers, heart problems, asthma problems, colon problems, and depression. Satan was winning me very fast and the worse thing about it all is I didn't care anymore. My doctors told me that I had a serious growth inside my abdomen and that it may be malignant. My greatest support system (my parents) was gone. I had nowhere to turn and nobody to turn to. As clear as the words I'm writing, my mother came to me in my sleep and said, "Remember from whence you came." I was up most of the night trying to figure out the meaning of her words. She and my Dad had always told me I was a special gift from God, for you see she had 5 miscarriages before God's gift of adoption.

By morning I was on my knees praying, "Help me Lord, I am back and I am sorry," praying for forgiveness for straying, for losing focus of the faith that really never went away but became so painful to admit. In spite of my actions and things I had said and done, my God told me all was forgiven and that He never left me nor had

He forsaken me. As I walked down the center isle behind each of my parents' caskets it was Him that held my hand and massaged my unsteady heartbeat. (Psalms 34:4 - I sought the Lord and He answered me; He delivered me from all of my fears.) He listened to my pain and anger filled heart and when the time was right He eased that pain as He continues to do today.

That morning after our talk, as I rose from my knees, God welcomed me back into His comforting arms as a sheep of His flock. More importantly, I placed Him back in the driver's seat of my life. My GOD IS SUCH AN AWESOME GOD!!! He helped me find my biological family which includes one brother and three sisters establishing a new support system, brought me through a 20 year military career and 13 major operations, and provided for me new Christian friends in the Scott Inspirational Choir, and O'Fallon First Baptist Church. My God is such AN AWESOME GOD. (Psalms 34:8 - Taste and see that the Lord is good; blessed is the man who takes refuge in Him).

You see you can never forget from whence you came. Sometimes you can ignore what you know is right, but you don't forget it. My family is dwindling down to a few and the few that are left remain close. We count on each other and pray for each other knowing that family bonds make tough heart strings.

On the day of my mother's funeral my office in Oklahoma called me to let me know that I finally got orders to move to St. Louis and could be with my husband. On such a very sad day for me, I smiled. God knew I would be a mess if I had to go back and live alone, separated again from my dear husband. I did not share many of the feelings I expressed in that letter to my husband. I didn't think he would understand what was happening with me. Just being with him, living in the same home provided the support and love I needed.

He is an "On-time God." My family and I grow closer every day if there is such a thing. We still have lemons in our life but they are only sweetening the lemonade. My Aunt Josephine is 92 years blessed and she calls and prays for me just like I am one of her children. My "sister" Rhonda hops a plane every time I say, "I have to have surgery." My husband's cousins call me weekly and will hop a plane in a minute. My third and fourth (generation) cousins still call me often and come visit. I couldn't make lemonade out of life's lemons if I did not have family support. Thank God for them all.

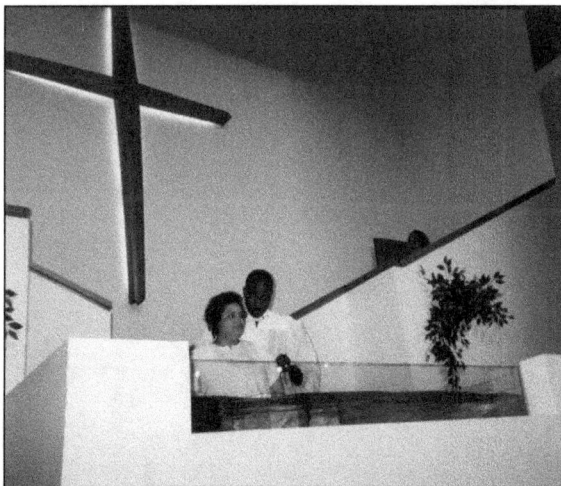

My Rededication Baptism with Bishop Dudley 2002

In 2002, I wanted to rededicate my life to Christ. I think in some way I was still saying I'm sorry for the wrong I have done, deserting you, losing my faith, and straying from my beliefs. But I wanted to put God back in the driver's seat of my life. I talked with my Pastor, Bishop Geoffrey Vincent Dudley. I asked if I could be baptized again. I explained I grew up Methodist and he knew their procedure. He told me he would do the baptizing. I told him I was young when I was baptized and that I was much wiser and spirituality had grown. I didn't tell him the rest of the reason.

On June 2, 2002 I rededicated my life to Christ with a submersion. Ok, now I know what my mom was talking about when she said a big tub with cold holy water. It wasn't a tub, but the water was cold. After being submersed instantly I felt warm. God's love is so comforting.

Reading Scripture

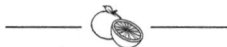

———— ⬭ ————

Reading the Holy Bible and receiving God's Word has been the central focus of my healing.

More recently than in the past I have asked myself, "Are you worthy of the mercy God has shown you?" I get many compliments on how inspiring my actions and attitude to the events I have been through are. I truly believe your attitude will help you through many things. On the days when I felt a moment of energy it was very easy for me to say I can beat "this" (whatever this was). But on the days when I was completely drained it was not easy to smile back when others smiled at me. The compliments people pay me actually inspire me as well.

What others say to us and what we say to ourselves can have such an impact. Filling my spirit and soul with Scripture has helped get me through. I read them sometimes 10 to 15 times a day. I share some of my favorites and hope they will help you too.

Family

Honor your father and your mother, that your days may be long upon the land which the Lord your God is giving you. Exodus 20:12

For this reason I bow my knees to the Father of our Lord Jesus Christ, from whom the whole family in heaven and earth is named... Ephesians 3:14-15

Wives, submit to your own husbands, as to the Lord. Ephesians 5:22

Husbands, love your wives, just as Christ also loved the church and gave Himself for her… Ephesians 5:25

Children, obey your parents in the Lord, for this is right. Ephesians 6:1

And you, fathers, do not provoke your children to wrath, but bring them up in the training and admonition of the Lord. Ephesians 6:4

Faith

… the just shall live by his faith. Habakkuk 2:4

Then the disciples came to Jesus privately and said, "Why could we not cast it out?" So Jesus said to them, "Because of your unbelief; for assuredly, I say to you, if you have faith as a mustard seed, you will say to this mountain, 'Move from here to there,' and it will move; and nothing will be impossible for you. However, this kind does not go out except by prayer and fasting. Matthew 17:19-20

But without faith it is impossible to please Him, for he who comes to God must believe that He is, and that He is a rewarder of those who diligently seek Him. Hebrews 11:6

Trust in the LORD WITH ALL YOUR HEART, And lean not on your own understanding; In all your ways acknowledge Him, And He shall direct your paths. Proverbs 3:5-6

- Jo Ann Speer Martin

Inspiration

But there is a spirit in man: and the inspiration of the Almighty giveth them understanding. Job 32:8

The spirit of God hath made me, and the breath of the Almighty hath given me life. Job 33:4

I can do all things through Christ who strengthens me. Philippians 4:13

Trust in the LORD WITH ALL YOUR HEART, And lean not on your own understanding; In all your ways acknowledge Him, And He shall direct your paths. Proverbs 3:5-6

Oh, taste and see that the LORD IS GOOD; Blessed is the man who trusts in Him! Psalm 34:8

The righteous cry out, and the Lord hears, And delivers them out of all their troubles. The Lord is near to those who have a broken heart, And saves such as have a contrite spirit. Psalm 34:17-18

… and that from childhood you have known the Holy Scriptures, which are able to make you wise for salvation through faith which is in Christ Jesus. 2 Timothy 3:15

Healing

Your word is a lamp to my feet, And a light to my path. Psalm 119:105

Your testimonies I have taken as a heritage forever, For they are the rejoicing of my heart. Psalm 119:111

My son, give attention to my words; Incline your ear to my sayings. Do not let them depart from your eyes; Keep them in the midst of your heart; For they are life to those who find them, And health to all their flesh. Proverbs 4:20-22

Worship the Lord your God, and his blessing will be on your food and water. I will take away sickness from among you, and none will miscarry or be barren in your land. I will give you a full life span. Exodus 23:24-26, NIV

My Life In Pictures...

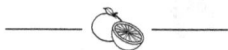

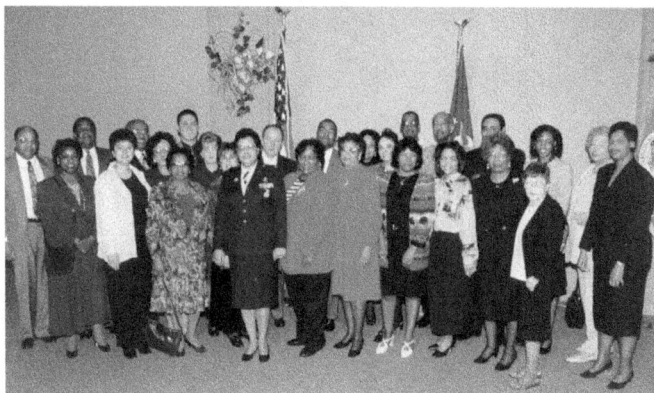

30 Family Members from Around the World Jo Ann's Retirement
Celebration 1998

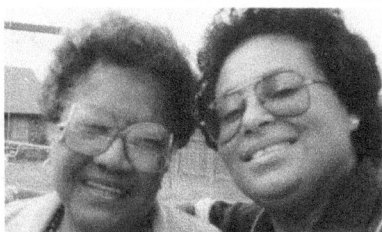

Mom and Daughter

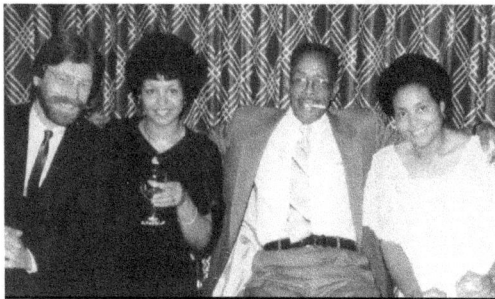

Elmar, Peggy, My Dad James and Me

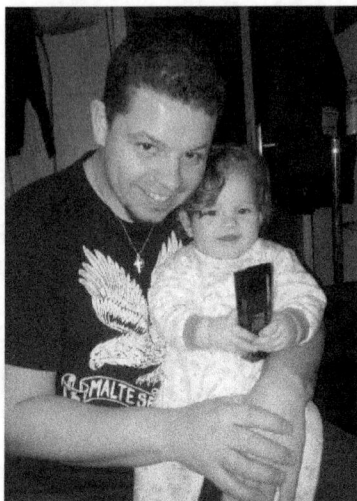

Nephew Michael with His Daughter Sophia

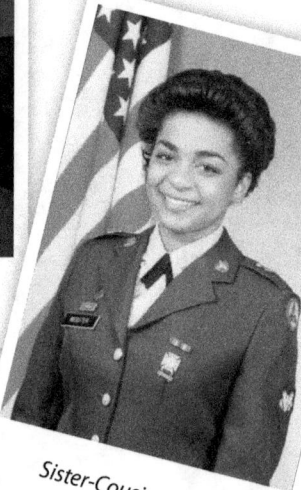

Sister-Cousin Rhonda

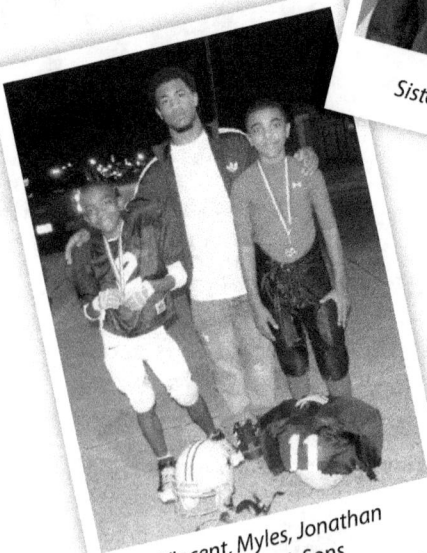

Vincent, Myles, Jonathan -Rhonda's Sons

- Jo Ann Speer Martin

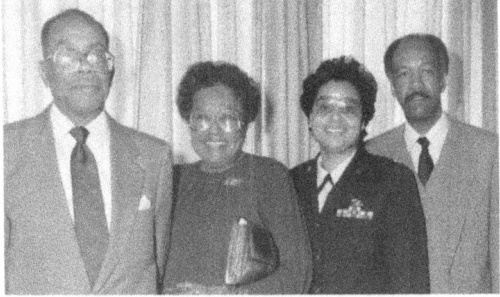

My First Commander's Reception Dad, Mom,
Me and Marty

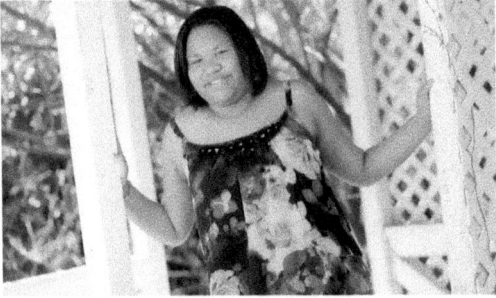

My God Daughter Rayna Campbell

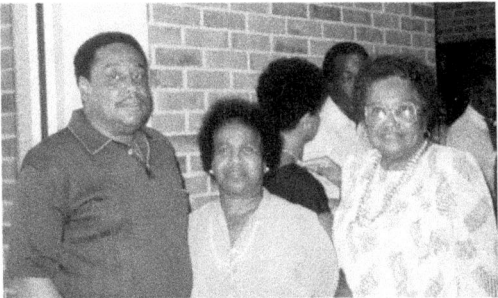

My God Parents, John & Catherine Williams with My
Mom Helyn

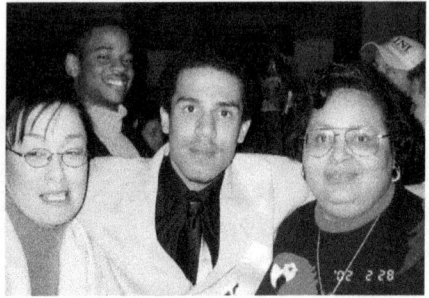

My God Son Nao, His Mom Aki and Me

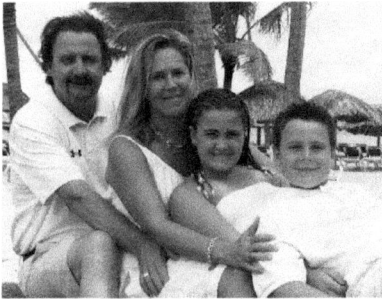

My Niece Anne (Hugh) and Her Family

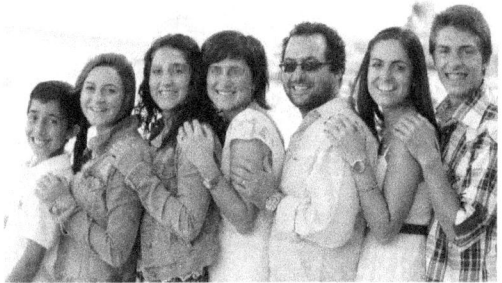

My Niece Monica (Paul) and Family

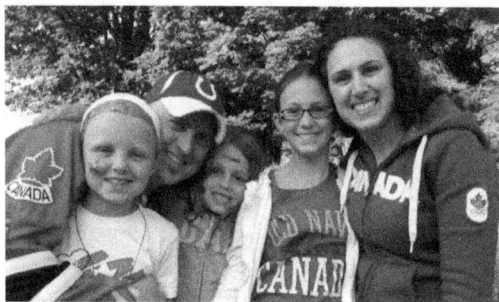

My Niece Petra (Kirk) and Her Family

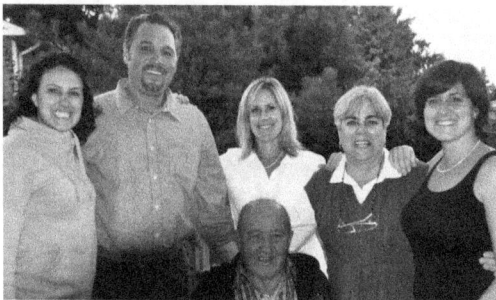

*Petra, John, Anne, Rosie (My Sister-in-Law), Monica
and My Brother Peter (Seated)*

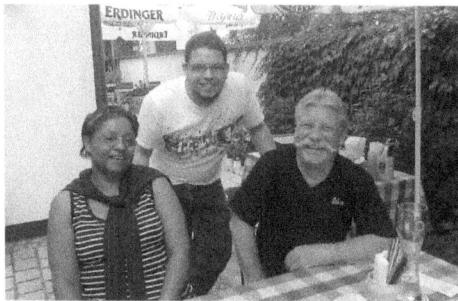

Sister Peggy and Elmar Schwab with Son Michael

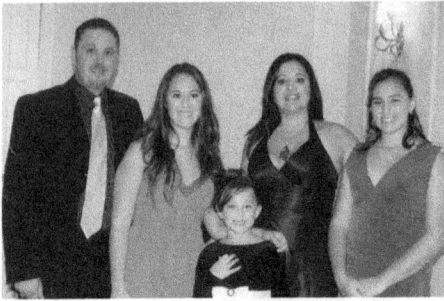

My Nephew John (Christine) Family

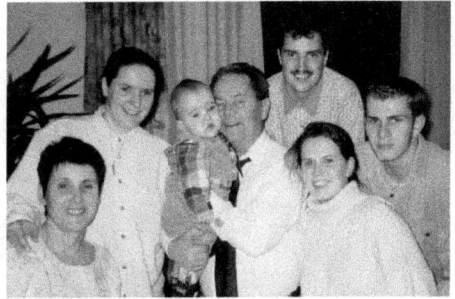

The Pape Family

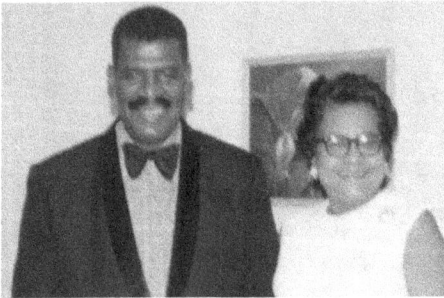

Uncle Al & Aunt Florence

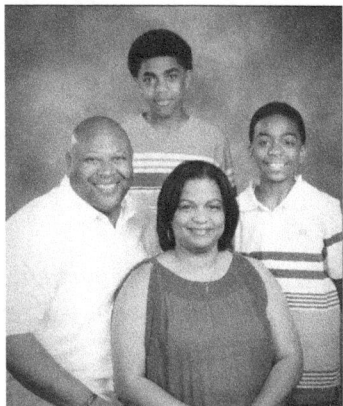

Clifton and Rhonda with Vincent and Jonathan (Myles not Pictured)

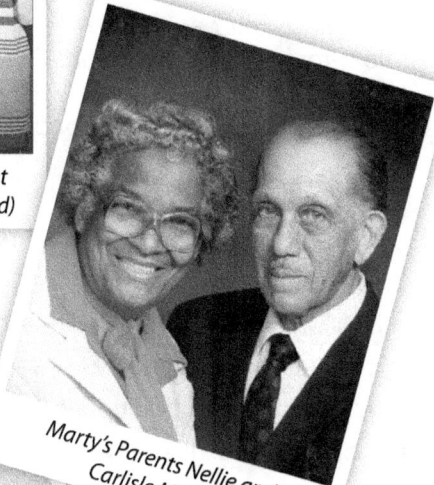

Marty's Parents Nellie and Carlisle Martin

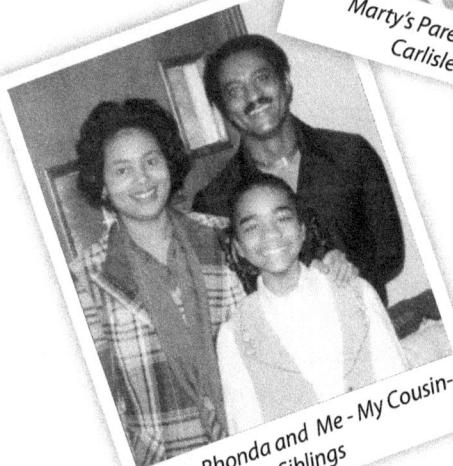

Mike, Rhonda and Me - My Cousin-Siblings

Tonsillitis, Bronchitis and Appendicitis???

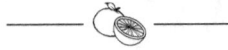

Moses told the people of Israel, "And the Lord, He it is that doth go before thee; He will be with thee, He will not fail thee, neither forsake thee; fear not neither dismay.
Deuteronomy 31:6-8

For as long as I can remember, I have been in and out of doctor's offices. At a young age I had tonsillitis all the time. If it wasn't tonsillitis, it was bronchitis. Then one day while I was in high school, I woke up with a pain in my side. It hurt really badly, but I loved school and knew if I said something to my parents they would probably keep me home. I got dressed and caught the bus as usual. It seemed to me the bus hit every pot hole in the street on the way to school and by the time I got there I was really in pain. I went directly to the principal's office and told him I was really hurting. He called my mom at work and sent me to the nurse's office. It wasn't very long before I heard heels coming down the hall so fast, it sounded like someone was running. I knew that was my mom.

She helped me to the car because by then I was doubled over. Off to the doctor's office we went. We didn't have an appointment, but we only had a 15-minute wait before we were called back. The doctor took one look at me, poked me in the stomach and said I needed surgery because my appendix

- Jo Ann Speer Martin

needed to be removed. The look on my mother's face alone scared me to death. The next thing I know, they were calling my dad and told him to meet us at the hospital. That was my first ambulance ride. If I hadn't been in so much pain, it might have been fun. There was so much in that truck to look at. It was a short ride because the doctor's office and the hospital were not that far apart.

When we got there mom, registered me and the nurses began an IV for me. I looked up. Dad had gotten there and was standing in the hall talking with mom. They both came in and told me I was about to have stomach surgery for my appendix and I would be just fine. They could not go with me, but would see me when it was over. The nurses rolled my bed down the hall. One put a shot into the IV and that is about all I remember. I woke up in a hospital room with mom and dad right there holding my hand. My mom was saying, "Thank you Lord," when I opened my eyes. Dad told me my appendix had ruptured and I was a sick child but after a day or two I would be okay. At this point in my life, it was not my most foremost thought to stop and thank God for saving me, not even after hearing my mom say, "Thank you Lord." I thought you thanked the Lord when you said your prayers at night before going to bed. My spiritual life has grown tremendously since then. Little did I know this would be the first of many times I would be in the hospital.

Breathing and My Body

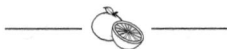

But He was wounded for our transgressions, He was bruised for our iniquities: the chastisement of our peace was upon Him; and with His stripes we are healed. Isaiah 53:5

By 1983, I had undergone many surgeries; appendix removed, lesions off my eye, moles on the back of my neck, several laparoscopes on my stomach for endometriosis, an ovarian cyst removed, bleeding ulcers, a broken foot, and a severed Achilles. Fortunately for me none of these things were malignant. They were all benign, but the surgeries had taken a toll on my body. I had now developed asthma, which I had never had before. I was in the service now and that meant there were a lot of physical things I was required to do in order to stay fit. I never had a waiver for any of those things, but asthma definitely made it hard to continue passing the fitness tests. I managed though, by calling on the Lord many times.

My asthma seemed to get worse every year and I was spending more and more time in the hospital for asthma attacks. I had a bout of pneumonia for the first time in 1984. As a result, if I caught a cold or had bronchitis, I was really sick. My doctor prescribed a drug called prednisone, which helped my asthma, but it had so many side effects. I gained weight and I became an insulin-dependent diabetic. One day, I was tired of how the side effects were having an effect on me and I stopped taking the

- Jo Ann Speer Martin

medicine. That was a mistake because I landed in the hospital. The doctor told me I could learn to be fat and happy or skinny and dead. What a choice. I could choose happiness or death. I wasn't ready to die, so I got back on the medicine.

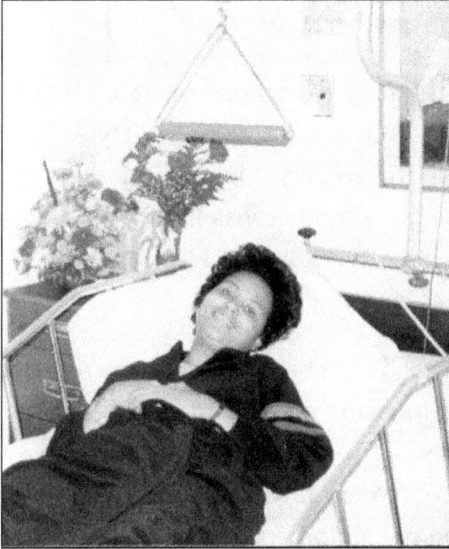

Me in a Hospital Bed

Once I got back on the medicine, it became harder and harder for me to pass my physicals for the Air Force. I had weight standards to meet. Two weeks before my physicals, I would have to starve myself so I could make weight. I would also sit in the sauna for an hour, run a mile and go back to the sauna before running to go get weighed. I made it until my retirement in 1998. I know that would not have been possible without God in my life and the encouragement and support from my parents and friends.

My next scare was in 1992. I was playing racquetball and twisted my knee. I did a lot more than twist my knee; I actually tore the meniscus, rearranged the patella and severed the right ACL. I had to have orthoscopic surgery. The surgeon said they could fix everything except my ACL that was severed. Fixing the ACL would require another surgery.

I scheduled the surgery to repair my ACL. I was an athlete and not having my ACL was cramping my style. The week before I was to have the surgery, I lost my mother. I cancelled the surgery. Losing my mother was hard on me because my dad had passed in 1991, but I knew I was not alone because I had the support of family.

To this day I still do not have an ACL in my right leg, I never got it repaired. A lot of my "get up and go" was now gone. I decided when I hit the 20 year mark in the Air Force, I would retire. During my retirement physical, the Air Force doctor found a huge mass in my abdomen. They thought it was Cancer and sent me to Barnes Hospital in St. Louis, Missouri for surgery. It was an intense surgery and I ended up having to have a complete hysterectomy and had not yet given birth to children.

I remember the bible saying be fruitful and even today that is a touchy subject with me. Every since I can remember I have always wanted children. When I was young I use to want ten. My dad would always joke with me and say, "Well don't bring them here." I was not blessed to have children but was blessed to share other people's children. I am always saying to my husband, we can take this one home with us. The parents always laugh and reply, "But you will bring them back before midnight."

- Jo Ann Speer Martin

I was fairly healthy for about 2 years and one night while my husband was playing cards in the basement with his friends, a pain hit me in the chest. I thought I was having a heart attack. Immediately I told him, "You have to stop and take me to the emergency room." All the card players jumped up and left. Off to the hospital we went. This was when Scott AFB still had an emergency room. The doctor took one look at me and said, "Colonel Martin you will need to have surgery, it's your gallbladder." I wasn't convinced. You know some doctors are ready to operate on a hang nail. He had only taken blood, blood pressure, and my temperature. How could he know this?

He could tell I didn't believe him. He said, "I am going to admit you and do a test in the morning for your benefit before surgery." The next morning I went for the test. They used some kind of dye which my gall bladder was supposed to absorb in so many minutes. Needless to say my gall bladder failed the test miserably. So once again I was going under the knife.

Before the surgery, I informed the surgeon about the adhesions in my abdomen from previous surgeries. The surgeon decided to do a laser surgery instead of the normal surgery. The surgery was longer than normal, but God was holding my hand and guiding the hand of the surgeon. I was back in the swing of things in a week. But the adhesions are beginning to cause additional problems for me.

Carotid Artery/Strokes

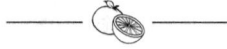

On June 10, 2011, while working at my church on the computer all at once I went blind. I told my co-worker, Dave, that I could not see.

He asked me, "Can't see what?"

I replied, "I can't see anything."

He was ready to call an ambulance. I begged him to please just wait a minute. I was not in any pain, but the fear of going blind was frightening. In about 15-20 minutes my sight started to come back. At first, it was like I was looking at a photo negative and then my sight returned. I had no idea what had just happened, but I made an appointment to see my eye doctor.

She checked my eyes and they were fine. She recommended I see my regular doctor. I made the appointment with the doctor and after listening to the arteries in my neck, he wanted me to see another type of eye doctor. I did that as well. That eye doctor told me I needed to see a vascular doctor. Before I could see the vascular doctor, my husband's mother, Momma Nellie, passed in Virginia. Off to Virginia we went. While in Virginia for the funeral it happened again. I went completely blind. This time it was for only about 15 minutes. Once we returned from the funeral, I made a new appointment with the vascular doctor,

- Jo Ann Speer Martin

but it would be a while before I would be able to see the doctor, Dr. Hans Moosa. During the time before my appointment, I was still working and driving. When I saw the doctor, he did a battery of tests and discovered I had three mini strokes which they call TIAs which left no lasting effects, but I would need surgery because my carotid artery was 93 percent blocked and it needed cleaning out. Dr. Moosa told me there was a slight chance I could have a stroke on the table. There was an 85 percent chance of having a massive stroke in 12 months if I didn't have the surgery. There were no questions in my mind. This is what I was going to do. God is GREAT!

He told me that the surgery was very serious because it is on an artery and there is a chance it will cause a stroke, but it is a very common surgery. I prayed as many of my friends and family did, even strangers prayed for my well-being. I hoped that God would continue to allow me to do his work here on earth. The day of the surgery came and after much prayer, I was ready.

I don't know how long surgery lasted, but it was longer than normal. When I woke up, I had a huge bandage all the way down the side of my face and I hurt pretty badly. I thought to myself after all the surgery I have had, this feels like more than four inches. I slept off and on that day and the next morning the nurses came in to remove the bandages. I looked in the mirror and was just shocked. I had an 11 inch hideous scar that went from behind my ear, down my neck to the front at my collarbone. It was full of staples just like you use on paper.

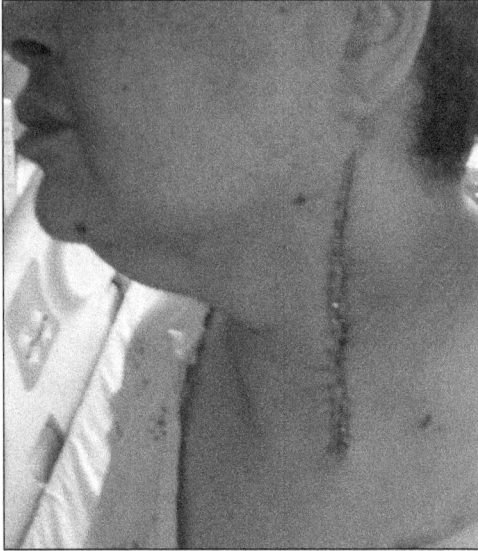

Surgery Two

The doctor came in and explained how blessed I was. You are supposed to have a "Y" in your artery about three inches below your ear. Dr. Moosa explained my scar was so long because my "Y" was under my collar bone. He had to search for it. He wasn't bragging, but said a less experienced doctor may have had a completely different outcome. We all know what doctor was really in charge. God has walked into every operating room with me and held my hand. He not only holds hands but guides the thoughts of the doctors and their hands. Isn't He awesome? I have not had a TIA (mini stroke) since the surgery two years ago. I just had my check up and all is well in my arteries.

Chrons Disease

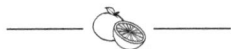

With as much as I went through in 2011, I thought 2012 would be the year I didn't have to see a hospital. It turned out to be a year I would never forget. I had been very ill with a disease called Chrons, which is a form of inflammatory bowel disease. In 2012, I had been very ill because of the disease, but I was diagnosed with it in 2004. This was the worse and longest attack I have ever had. I had lost over 100 pounds in about seven months. After many doctor visits and five hospital trips, I decided that the surgery all the doctors spoke of was right around the corner. So, I started to research where to have it, which surgeon should do it, etc. I had it all planned out and the week before I was to meet with my new doctor, I was put in the hospital. I would not allow surgery that night and requested that the surgery be done at Barnes because of my extensive surgery history and I had already picked out a doctor and surgeon at Barnes. The next morning, an ambulance took me to Barnes and I met a surgeon, not the one I picked. This surgeon was also the professor that taught doctors at Barnes how to do the surgery I was about to have. That is when I realized God had taken over my plans and put His in the works.

The surgeon talked with my husband and me and from the pictures and tests was very sure that I would have a colostomy bag after surgery. To prepare for surgery I had to have a colonoscopy, but I was not able to have one done and ended up having the surgery without that procedure.

Prior to my surgery, I talked with the Bishop of my church and explained what they were about to do to me and before he prayed he told me "sometimes man has a good plan but God has better plan", he assured me we were praying for God's plan, no colostomy bag.

My surgery was extremely long. Although I was in a lot of pain while in recovery, the nurse reports I continued to say "Thank You Lordy," out loud for so long other patients in the room started saying it also. I thought that was funny.

I was in recovery so long they let Marty and my cousin, Rhonda, whom I have always referred to as my sister, come back for a minute. I kept feeling my stomach for the colostomy bag and when Marty came in he leaned over and told me, "Baby you did not have to have the bag. They just removed the bad intestines". Oh what an awesome God we serve! They removed 35 inches of my small intestine and I am back to eating regular food. Praise God! Praise God for His plan. God always knows best. He never left me. In fact He continues to hold my hand today as I continue to recuperate. To God be all the glory.

Little did I know what was around the corner. I was in the hospital for 15 days and released. Recuperating fine, and a month later, my stomach busted open in my kitchen. I hollered for Marty and off to the ER in St Louis we went.

The doctors said I had an abscess under my incision and could not have known other than the pain. I had been having pain, but I thought it was part of my recuperation. Back in the hospital I went. When I got out this time, I had a nurse come to my house three times a week.

The doctors did not want me using my intestines, so they wanted me to get a feeding tube. In seven months, I went from size 22 to size 8. Now I am having problems with the feeding tube and I have to have more surgery. As a result of this surgery, I now have massive blood clots in my neck. Until this gets regulated, I have to see my doctor every two weeks and take a new medicine.

Because of the location of the clots, I cannot lay flat in a bed or my face and eyes swell up to the point that my eye closes. SOOOO I am sleeping sitting up in a chair. It still swells but not as much.

Because of His Mercy and Goodness I am Still Here Praising My Lord

Believe me when I tell you there were many days in 2012 that I questioned my faith in God. How could I be afraid of going to surgery if my faith in God was strong? I never asked the question, "Why me?" I just continued to tell myself that I am special and God chose me because somehow, through Him we could handle what I was going through. I knew there was a reason and writing this book may have been the reason. I never really wanted to write a book but I do know that I have read some books that truly gave me inspiration when I needed it. During my hospital stay, I looked around at those that were sicker than I was and was reminded how blessed I really am. I want others to know they can also find healing through belief and faith in God. When life throws you a curve look around at the curves in other's life and know you are blessed.

Chrons disease is a serious monster and I didn't really know how bad it was until I started to have long attacks. Sometimes these attacks would last for months. During my last Chrons attack that lead to the surgery and I lost 130 pounds. My friends looked at me like I was going to die any second. That wasn't really bad though; it's when total strangers who never saw you at 230 pounds look at you like you are a very ill person is when it sinks in that you are sick. I was really weak after being in the bed so long then the surgery. I used to pray, "God if you help me lose some weight..." I didn't think I would have to get sick to lose the weight. So, be careful what you ask God for, He helped me lose some weight alright. It was the prayers and support of family and friends that gave me the courage to continue to try and come back to being strong. I truly believed God in His time would bring me back to all the foods I loved and heal my stomach. So many times I wanted to just give up and then I would think of all the encouragement and God's promises. I would think how others were counting on me to pull through this and realize giving up was not an option. It was a long recovery for me but it was worth it.

Chrons is not something you want your worst enemy to have, but some good things came from that experience. After years of dieting, I was back to my high school weight and although my present friends had not seen me this size, it really made me smile. I joke with my husband to look out because I am back to my "high school fine." Not only that, I got a new wardrobe.

One of the best things is my blood pressure is back to normal and I am off my medication for it. *I am no longer diabetic.* I don't have to take any shots or pills for diabetes anymore. I still take my blood sugar every now and then to keep check, but oh what a blessing this is.

With all of my different illnesses, I was taking 32 pills a day. I am now down to eight. I know eight sounds like a lot, but when you came from 32, eight is not so bad. This is just one of many testimonies of how God has blessed my life.

Breast Cancer

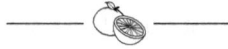

———— 🍊 ————

Well, 2012 was just about over and I was anxiously awaiting a healthy 2013. I was not quite well from the Chrons surgery when I had my regular mammogram. I'll get right to the point, after three mammograms, an MRI, and a biopsy, I was told I have breast Cancer. This is major surgery three years in a row and one of the reasons I am writing this book.

I received a call in March 2013 from my doctor to make an appointment so he could go over my test results. When I got the call, I just knew it was going to be good news. Marty and I went to the appointment and the receptionist said that Marty could go in the back with me. Now every other time I had been there for tests, they said he had to stay in the waiting room. The fact he could go with me started me to thinking this may not be good. As we walked down the hall the nurses spoke to me but not with that great big smile I was used to seeing. They led us to the waiting area and closed the door. The doctor and one nurse who was with me during the biopsy came in and sat down. The doctor was right in front of me and the nurse right beside me with Marty on the other side of me.

The doctor spoke to us both and looked me right in the eyes and said, "Colonel Martin the news is not good. You have breast Cancer."

- Jo Ann Speer Martin

The words alone took about five seconds to sink in and I looked up at Marty when he dropped his head. Instantly and totally involuntarily, the tears started to flow from eyes. No matter how hard I tried not to cry they would not stop. I had not said a word but the doctor continued to talk. I really did not hear anything he said for the next five minutes. At this point I really wanted to say, "Why me Lord?" but with all that I had been through, I was past asking that.

I said to my doctor, "You know why I have this now? Because God knows I can handle it."

The nurse got up to get tissues and when she returned her eyes were as red as I am sure mine were. I wondered if the tissue was for me or for her. Well, in five minutes my mind went everywhere. At minute six, the time was up for my pity party. I looked at my husband and said, "Are you ready to fight?" He nodded his head and gave me a slight yet confident smile. With God, together, we would make it.

The doctor explained the next steps and asked if I had any questions. For a person who always has questions, I had none at that moment. I apologized for crying and was told it is a normal reaction, not to apologize. We all stood up and Marty said, "Let's go start this fight." As we left the doctor told me, "Col. Martin, Cancer does not mean death."

As I write this book while going every day to radiation therapy – CANCER FREE, I am a living witness with millions of others that Cancer does not mean death. God is not through with me.

Marty and I went to the Siteman Cancer Center at Barnes Hospital to see an oncology surgeon about my options. On the way, I prayed that God would help me make the right decision. I had already decided I wanted a complete mastectomy because I didn't want to deal with this again. I also wanted to get my husband's opinion about what I should do.

He said, "Your health right now is not very good and you have really been through a lot, so I feel like you should have a lumpectomy."

At least now I knew his true feelings. I wanted a complete mastectomy and Marty wanted me to have a lumpectomy, but I didn't know God's plan.

The doctor gave us a 200-page book to read while we were in the office and left us alone to read it. I opened the book to scan and the first page I turned to said that most people think once they have a mastectomy, Cancer will not reappear in that breast and that is not true. I began to feel God speaking to me. I flipped to another page and there it said having a lumpectomy and radiation is 100% as effective as a mastectomy, depending on the size of the Cancer. I am hearing God loud and clear now and I change my mind at that moment to have a lumpectomy. The doctor agreed with my decision.

When you show up for surgery there are a few steps to the process. You do all the paperwork in one place. Then you go and have blood drawn in another place. Next, you have nuclear medicine placed in your breast to light it up for the doctor to see. If anyone tells you to go to Nuclear Medicine, turn around and RUN in the opposite direction. I was not numbed for this process and they use a huge needle. Oh, and most important, don't move or they have to do it over again.

Then I headed to another place to have four mammograms done. I am in pain from being given the nuclear medicine and now they want to put my breast in the breast vice. After that, they have metal markers and a wire placed in the breast to guide the doctor during surgery. At least I had a small amount of numbing medicine for this procedure. All of this was done while I was awake. I thought for sure I was not going to be awake for this part, but I was wrong. I was in so much pain and I had had enough, but I still had to get an IV. A nurse tried earlier, but could not get it started. *At this point, I am ready to be knocked out for surgery.*

A new nurse is going to put my IV in, but she is having a hard time as well.

I asked her, "Are you alright? You are really sweating and it is cold in here."

She replied, "Mrs. Martin, when nurses can't get IVs started on patients like you, they call me. I am good and I can't get your IV started."

I apologized and she assured me it was not my fault. I have always been what they call, "a hard stick." I grabbed her hand and said a short prayer and when I finished, she said, "Amen." On the next try, she got the vein and the IV was running well.

We both smiled and thanked God at the same time.

I asked her, "What's next?"

She said, "Surgery." The anesthesiologist came in the room with another man and I asked if I could get the doctor and the nurse that would be with me in my room along with the three people that were already there. They all came in and I said a prayer.

Marty's cousin Lois, and Marty took care of me and called all the family to let them know the good news, the doctor thought he got all of the Cancer and did not think it was in my lymph nodes but would not be sure until pathology reports came back. While I am recovering at home, I find out I have the BRACA1/2 gene. I call it the "Angelina Jolie Test." I tell the doctor had I known this before surgery, I would have had a mastectomy. But that was not in God's plan. I am tired of having surgeries; I have had 18. No more.

In the meantime, I had to get my port put in for chemotherapy, yet another surgery. When I arrived at this place it was called, "Interventional Radiation." While the lady was typing all of my info into the computer I kept reading the sign behind her out loud, "Interventional Radiation." I said it so many times that the lady behind the desk started laughing.

I asked, "Why do they call it interventional radiation?"

She said she really did not know. My devotion for that morning talked about man listening to man when God is trying to speak. I had not connected the dots at this point though.

The doctor told Marty and I after the procedure that the veins in my chest were already collapsed and he could not insert the port. No chemo. My oncologist didn't want the port in my groin because of a risk of infection. Now I am wondering why it was recommended to have chemo any way. She explained to me that chemo is given to decrease the chance of having the Cancer return, but some people who have had chemo see the Cancer return. I understood clearly. The decision was made to only have radiation.

As I write this book, I go to radiation every morning, Monday though Friday. The radiation makes me tired and always sleepy, but I am not in a lot of pain. I am so thankful for the blessings God affords me every day.

Choosing Life

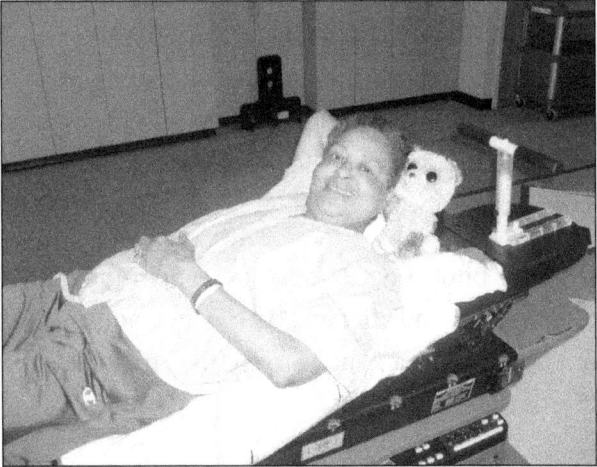

Jo Ann and Fam

When you have been extremely sick for basically three years and you are still on this side of the dirt, it has to be for a reason. I have chosen as my reasons; because I am special and because God has answered my prayer to allow me to spread the word of his goodness here on earth. So many days during the last three years I was in the type of pain that makes you want to give up on life.

Writing this book has not been easy for me during this time. I don't really think it would have been easy at any time because it took me down so many memory lanes. But friends and family have supported me all the way.

A friend whose husband had Cancer two years ago bought him a radiation buddy (which was a stuffed toy moose) to take with him when he went for treatment. The minute they found out about my Cancer they sent me "Fam." I have four family members who died from Cancer and I couldn't think of one name that was a combination of all of their names so I named my ewok "Fam" (short for family). Fam went with me to every radiation treatment. All the doctors and nurses know Fam now. Fam knows all of my deepest secrets and all of my fears, Fam prays with me, reads the Bible with me, and has really encouraged me in a 'Fam' kind of way. Fam doesn't talk much so I knew all of my secrets were safe. Because Fam helped so much to lighten the mental burden, I recommend everyone get their own ewok! I met a new friend while going to radiation and bought her a "Sofia." She brought her radiation buddy with her every day just like I did.

The Air Force and Beyond

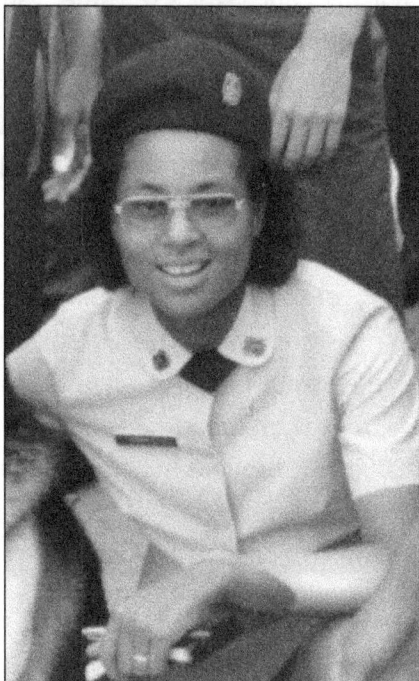

Jo Ann 1975 ROTC During Basic Training

I've shared so much about every other part of my life, this story would not be complete without including my work life. I am a hard worker, I like structure and I believe in good leadership. Some of the best times of my life happened either "at work" or "because of work." And, truth be told, being in the military is a way of life, not just work. God has blessed me with a wonderful military career.

- Jo Ann Speer Martin

In 1977, I graduated from Grambling State University where I was a part of the ROTC program. My father was a 27 year veteran of the United States Army. He retired as a Sergeant Major. Many of my friends were in the program and I knew the Commander, so I decided to join in my sophomore year. After joining, I learned I really enjoyed it. You have a command section to run just like you were in the service. Everyone had rank and you went through drills every week. You had inspections of your performance in whatever job you were assigned. There were real military personnel who trained you, kept you on track, and ran the detachment. I was in ROTC Detachment 311 two years and I don't think during that time my mother realized that meant when I graduated I would be going in the service and moving away from home. She was one hundred percent support until that little fact sunk in. The closer we got to graduation day the more she realized my time at home was short. The day of graduation I was also commissioned in the United States Air Force as a Second Lieutenant. You know I was looking sharp and crisp in my uniform. I think I shined my shoes for hours. My parents were so proud. I was getting my degrees and I was becoming an officer in the Air Force.

Michigan

My parents were so proud of me and I was too. They were very supportive of me. My first assignment was to K.I. Sawyer Air Force Base in Marquette, Michigan. I had to drive to the base, so my parents suggested my cousin, Mike, who was like my brother, go with me. Off we go.

The further north we go, the harder it snowed. I grew up in Louisiana and I had only seen snow twice in my life. This was very new to me to see so much snow. I am glad Mike is with me. We finally reach the base only to be told the base is closed because of the weather. So now we have to drive 20 miles back to Marquette in the very weather that closed the base to find a hotel for the night. I also had to let my sponsor, who helps recruits get settled on the base, know I had arrived, but could not get on base. The next day, I drop Mike off at the airport and I head to base to get settled.

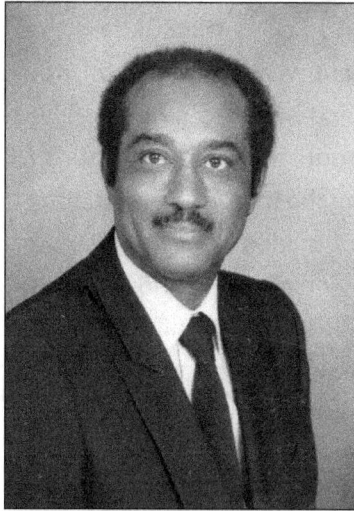

My Cousin-Brother Mike

I thought I was through with the snow, but that base gets an average of 80 inches of snow a year. We planned a barbeque for the Fourth of July. That morning it began to snow and in about an hour, there was 30 inches of snow on the ground. I had to call

- Jo Ann Speer Martin

my parents and tell them about this snow. I also learned why the buildings on the base are painted bright colors, so you can see them in white-out blizzards. In spite of all the snow, there were some days of great weather. I came to love the outdoors while in Michigan. I even bought a boat and a snowmobile.

While at the base, I was in the 87th Fighter Interceptor Squadron (The Red Bulls) as a Material Control Officer providing parts for B-52 Bombers, F-106 Fighter Jets and other training planes at the base. I had three other duties as well as an AV Fuels Officer, the War Readiness Material Officer and the Combat Turnaround Load Monitor.

I met a lot of people on the base who have become lifelong friends. Chief Master Sergeant, Thomas Tabor, who was nicknamed, "Terrible Tom Tabor" because of his most direct approach to everything. Tom was old enough to be my father and he took me under his wing and he kept me on the straight and narrow. He kept me out of trouble and taught me everything I knew at that time.

Two more people who became my "Best Friends Forever" were Captain Burl Hickman and his wife, Kathi. When I arrived at the base, this was my first time being away from home. Captain Hickman and his wife made my life much easier. Burl flew the planes I helped keep in the air. I learned a lot from both of them. They had two young children, Enith and Jonathan, and I became their babysitter. I became a part of their family, even going with them on family vacations.

Illinois

In 1982, I was assigned to the Headquarters Air Force Communications Command at Scott Air Force Base as an Inspector on the Inspector General Team. This was one of my best assignments. I was single and I got to travel around the world. While on this team, I was promoted to Captain and recommended for a below-the-zone promotion to Major. Going below-the-zone meant I was selected for this promotion a year before I was eligible to become a major. While on the team we traveled to England, Korea, Guam, Alaska, Australia, Hawaii, Japan, and many other countries but the most important for me was Germany.

It was while I was at Scott Air Force Base, that I met PeeWee and then Marty. My responsibilities were to inspect and brief the base officials prior to the inspection and upon our leaving. This was new and exciting for me as a young officer. I remember being on the other end making sure all the "i's were dotted and the t's crossed," getting ready for an inspection. When the team arrives there is a briefing given to the base officials and when the team leaves there is the briefing of everything that we found (good and bad) along with a rating for each major entity on base and an overall rating. This briefing goes along with a huge written report of everything briefed. I did the in and out briefings. I love to talk but when giving bad news to hundreds of people it really made me nervous. Funny I was nervous even when I was giving good news too. This assignment was without a doubt one of my favorite.

Germany

I was at Scott AFB for three years before I was assigned to Spangdahlem Air Base in Germany in 1985. I was assigned to the 52nd Supply Squadron as a Management and Systems Officer. This was a fun assignment. Germany is definitely a party place. There are so many places to visit and a festival for every occasion. Their stores close at 2pm on Saturday so if you are used to shopping all day on your off day you have to get up early. Germans generally shop on a daily basis for food. The refrigerators are small and they don't use freezers very much. It is even hard to get ice in a drink at dinner because most don't have freezers. Oh, but the food is awesome. I think I tasted everything they have to offer. Spangdahlem was up in the Eiffel Mountains so I had to drive a little bit to get to the bigger cities but I loved it. I made so many German friends while there and of course bonded with my biological mother PeeWee and my younger sister Peggy. This was the best part about the assignment. The other significant event during that time was getting married to Marty. I flew home got married and three days later, went back to work in Germany.

Indiana

My next assignment was at Grissom Air Force Base in Indiana. I was happy to be closer to Marty. While there, I was Chief of the Operations Support Branch and Acting Squadron Commander for the 305th Supply Squadron. I also joined the speaking team while I was there. The speaking team was established to speak to civilians about various topics when requested. Personally, I spoke to the Daughters of the American Revolution, among others. I really enjoyed doing that.

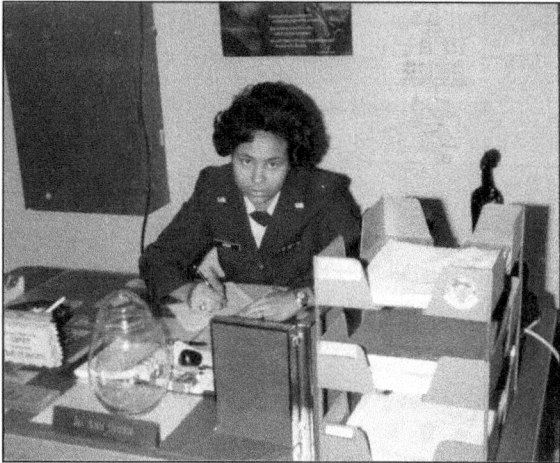

Jo Ann Hard at Work 1987

In this position there was a lot of paperwork and I wrote several operating procedures. It is also where I got my Commander's belt wet. I had never been a Commander although I had many officers and enlisted personnel under my supervision in the past. I could really tell at this point in my career that along with rank comes added responsibility. My Squadron was instrumental in the closure of the Howard Tanker Task Force in Panama and in the establishment of the Caribbean Tanker Task Force in Puerto Rico. In spite of the increased work and hours at this base I still managed to get my Master's Degree at Ball State University in Muncie, Indiana by going to night school. During this assignment I interacted with more high ranking base

- Jo Ann Speer Martin

officials and all of that was new for me. I learned more about giving respect and getting respect at this base than anywhere else. I matured quite a lot during this assignment and started to become a real leader, learning to fly on my own without having to be under someone else's wing. It started to become clear to me that along with rank and job position becoming a role model was also inevitable.

Oklahoma

In 1990 I was assigned to the 71st Air Base Group at Vance AFB in Enid, OK. You know I wasn't real happy to be going there because that made my commute about 9 ½ hours to see my husband. At Vance I had many jobs. I was the Chief of the Supply Management Division when I first arrived and that turned into the Logistics Squadron Commander. I was also the Assistant Deputy Base Commander on the Contingency Support Staff. My responsibilities included morale, welfare and recreation which was the bowling alley, library, golf course and a few others. Transportation, Supply, Mobility, and Civil Engineering also fell in my squadron. Vance's supply system was contracted out to a civilian entity and that was a first for me. One of my jobs was to provide surveillance over the performance of the contractor. I had a small military and civilian staff that if had they not been exceptional teachers and workers; I might have seen my first downfall. They taught me quickly about the ins and outs of my job. The contractors and I got along very well and I eventually gained everyone's respect for the knowledge I did have. That made things flow very well at Vance for me. I learned so much.

I also designed the 71st Logistics Squadron patch. While at Vance I lost my father to Cancer and my Mom to Diabetes. The loss of my father was really a blow that I know only God and my Mom got me through. But the loss of my Mom knocked all the wind out of my sails. When I left Vance I was really ready to go. My job performance at Vance rewarded me with a promotion to Lieutenant Colonel.

Home

I was finally able to be assigned close to my husband in 1993 and be able to live in the same house. What a blessing that was. I was assigned to the Defense Mapping Agency, now called the National Geospatial Agency in St. Louis as the Director of Logistics. This job proved to be challenging for me. I supervised a few military people, but mostly civilian workers. My responsibility was scattered all over St. Louis. We made maps for war and peacetime. We made classified and unclassified; black and white and color maps; air and land maps. We also provided the administrative supplies, transportation and vehicles, and storage needed to run all the locations. The Defense Mapping Agency had a huge mission. At the time I was deciding to retire, my boss wanted to promote me to Colonel. I was tempted to stay, but I knew retirement was best. It was a bitter sweet occasion.

Mostly because of the many outstanding staffs I had, I was afforded many accolades while in the Air Force. I received the Defense Meritorious Service Medal, Meritorious Service Medal,

Air Force Commendation Medal with three oak leaf clusters, Joint Meritorious Unit Award, Air Force Outstanding Unit Award with one oak leaf cluster, National Defense Ribbon, Overseas Long Tour Ribbon, Air Force Longevity Ribbon with four oak leaf clusters, Air Force Expert Marksmanship Ribbon with Dual Qualifications, Air Force Training Ribbon, and I was selected Officer of the Year in 1992, 1993 and 1994.

During my career I also had the opportunity to be actively involved in organizations and communities where I was assigned. I was the recipient of the President's National Association for Equal Opportunities in Education Award. In addition to being named Who's Who Among American Female Executives, Who's Who Among Black Colleges and Universities, also I am a member of the Tuskegee Airmen.

Post Air Force

After retirement, I took a few months off. I used that time to do house projects I had put off for long enough. One day, I woke up with a feeling of wanting to do more with my time and I decided to become a substitute teacher, which allowed me to pick the days I wanted to work. With this extra income, I could do some shopping because that's what I love to do. I also continued speaking around the country. At one point, I received a permanent substitute teaching position which meant I had to go to work every day, do grades and meet with the parents at parent/teacher conferences. One day I had a bad asthma attack because my room was not air conditioned and it was hot. My doctor told me I could not go back to work.

I became bored again and I got a job at First Baptist Church in O'Fallon, IL. It was not long before my asthma reared its ugly head and put me in the hospital. But at least this time, my office was air conditioned.

I felt restless yet again, so I got a job at the customer service counter at a local YMCA in my area. I had to leave this job, but thank goodness it was not due to health reasons. They instituted a new rule saying you could not use your cell phones while working. By this time, I had received my license to become a realtor and needed to be available to my clients. For the past 13 years, I have been a realtor.

God has always blessed me and I felt it at home and throughout my career.

"Blessed me" does not mean that I didn't have struggles and hard times, it means I survived them all successfully while God held my hand. Sometimes it seems when you are at your lowest points there are people that hold you there. They continue to talk about how bad things are for you and how sorry they feel for you. I sought out friends that were "upbeat." They would encourage me and tell me, "You can make it, hang in there." That's where I got the saying, "I'm hanging tough." I am teased for saying that all the time.

Being A Leader

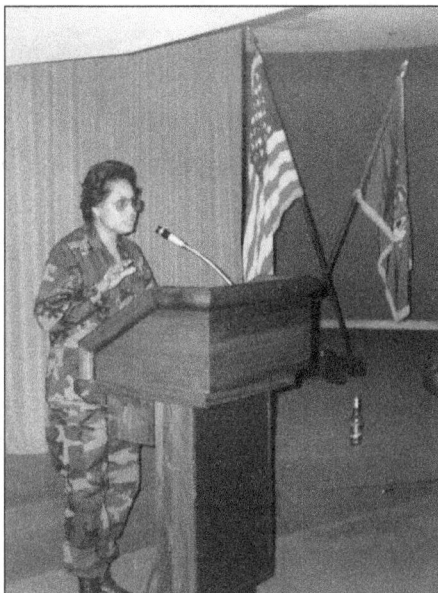

Jo Ann Speaking as a Commander

If you are going to be a leader, be the best leader you can be. That applies to anything you do. Don't be afraid to say, "I don't know," and ask for help. As you lead others, continue to remember how you would like to be lead. Mutual respect and appreciation build trust. Team and trust go a long way. Everyone has preferences and differences yet people appreciate guidance and clarity. Let everyone know what you expect up front and what the consequences are if you don't get it. There will be no surprises.

The Bitter and The Sweet

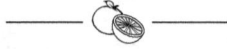

God never promised that things would be easy, but He always promised that He would never leave me or forsake me and He would go before me and prepare a place. He has held my hand through the easy walks of life and He's held it through the bad walks of life.

I wrote my obituary in 1998 because I was sick and I knew my husband could not do it. I was trying to protect those I would leave behind.

In a way that would be one sad thing they wouldn't have to go through, trying to dig up my life. While my sister-cousin Rhonda was here on the Fourth of July, I showed it to her, in the pink folder, its permanent home. I gave it to my sister, she read it. She took a deep breath and said, "Well, I'm glad to know you have actually done this."

I'm not trying to tell you I'm going to die. Marty is getting older and at least two people know it's here. It's kind of funny because Rhonda said, "I didn't know you minored in Chemistry." It is not written to the tune of an obituary, it is written to the tune of Ecclesiastes.

I don't see it as morbid because I have lived an absolutely blessed life despite everything which has happened to me.

- Jo Ann Speer Martin

It's morbid when you've had a lot of regrets about the life you lived or could have lived. It's morbid when it's with a sad heart or mind that it's written. I wasn't sad when I wrote it. I was happy I was very much alive when I wrote it.

I've always been told I am a real sentimentalist. Actually, I cry at the drop of a hat but don't like to admit it because I used to see crying as a sign of weakness. I've always had deep feelings and I just feel the need to look out for others.

When I think about my life, the only thing I probably would have done differently is to not smoke cigarettes. Sure, I eventually gave them up but, I would not have ever started if I could do it again.

Reflection

When I was in college I sat in on a riot and went to jail. I was only there for about three hours but I stood up for what I believed. It taught me many lessons. The biggest lesson being, I never want to be in jail. Because I wasn't afraid to speak my mind and stand up, I got in trouble. Was it worth it? I learned that I must pick which sword I want to fall on.

I had been in the service less than a year and punched a Colonel. I was a Second Lieutenant at the time. I thought my career was over but as it turned out, the Colonel had to apologize to me. Was it worth it? I learned there are certain lines which can't be crossed.

Always think ahead before opening your mouth or reacting. Every day try and inspire someone in some way. You never know how gentle gestures affect others.

Thank you for taking the time to learn a bit about my life.

Thinking about this journey reminds me of when I was in college. I would take my aunt Florida Jones and her friends, they were older than she, in their 70s, to the lake and fishing. They just loved getting in the car, riding out and then drinking beer, fishing and telling jokes. It was so funny especially because one of them was a preacher's mother. They got me once a month and I think I enjoyed it at least as much as they did. When I would drop them off they would say, "Jo Ann, thanks so much for taking time with us. We are old ladies and we just appreciate the time."

Time is a precious thing. Among the experiences and adventures, I truly treasure that precious gift from God. God Bless you and your family

As you move forward, treasure your gifts and your time.

Speaking of Time

In December of 1987 I was in the bed wearing a bathrobe and recovering from surgery when my sister Peggy called from Germany crying hysterically. "PeeWee passed away," she said. When I heard that I was devastated. Come to find out, she had a brain tumor. The news was hard to take. Bitter fruit. Yet, I was grateful for the few years we had together.

- Jo Ann Speer Martin

Life truly comes full circle. It is so ironic to be able to tell this story before going to print. Peggy got a phone call last month from a lady who introduced herself by saying, I am Tom Lacy's cousin and he made me promise to call this number for Peggy Loblein (Peggy's maiden name) before I left Germany. He has had this number since 1982 and did not know if it was still good. Peggy got really excited because she is the only one in my biological family that has actually met Tom. Tom Lacy drove me to meet my biological mother.

They talked for a while and Peggy couldn't wait to call me because we had just discussed Tom the week before. She said, "You will never guess who found me! Tom Lacy."

Of course then I got excited and asked, "Where is he?" She said, "He is in Bangkok. I have his e-mail address."

She sent it to me and I immediately wrote him a note. Within an hour he wrote me back. We have both been looking for each other since 1982.

The young lady I used to tease him about marrying is now his wife of 27 years. We will never lose touch again. We really have a lot to catch up on. I started this book with mental thoughts of the day I met PeeWee and how Tom stuck by me. I am finishing this book with finally finding the guy that made it all possible just by caring.

Refreshment

There is refreshed hope around every corner, if we hang in there long enough to look around that corner. You can't have sweet lemonade without a few bitter lemons, so when life deals you lemons – add your sugar, make lemonade and enjoy it enough to go out and inspire others.

- Jo Ann Speer Martin

A Note from the Publisher

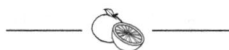

Mission Possible Press...

Creating Legacies through Absolute Good Works

As a publisher, I have the opportunity to transform hopeful writers into successful authors. This brings me great pleasure because I believe everyone has wisdom to share and valuable stories to tell.

Have you ever met a person and thought, "Whew, she/he reminds me of someone I know really well?" Well, Jo Ann Martin is one such person, for me at least. She is focused, determined, tough, a true leader and a mushy creampuff with a huge heart, all at the same time.

Helping her tell her stories and share her amazing experiences has been a life-changing, motivating experience. Why? Because she willed herself to LIVE until the very least, her book was complete. She does not let fear or circumstance deter her. She prays and prays to make it through, healing every step of the way. *Goodness, she has a storehouse of blessings to share for years to come.*

I am honored and pleased to present this book, *My Life's Lemonade, The Bitter and the Sweet,* written by Jo Ann Speer Martin as part of our Extraordinary Living Series.

In the Spirit of Communication,
Jo Lena Johnson,
Founder and Publisher
Mission Possible Press, A division of Absolute Good
www.AbsoluteGood.com
www.MissionPossiblePress.com

About the Author

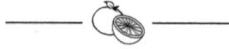

Jo Ann Speer Martin was born in Wurzburg, Germany, and naturalized as a United States citizen by her parents when her military father returned to the states. She was baptized as a Christian in the Lewis Temple C.M.E. Church in Grambling, LA., at the age of ten years old. She loved singing in the choir and going to church. She was not fond of Sunday School and didn't like how early it was. Her mom said, "No Sunday School, no playing today with your friends," so Jo Ann was *up and at'em,* every Sunday morning.

At a very young age she had health problems, but she didn't always know that Jesus could fix them if she asked Him. She grew up in a God-loving family, went to school and studied hard; graduated from Grambling High School, Grambling State University with her Bachelor's Degree in Biology and Chemistry, and Ball State University with her Master's Degree in Executive Development.

While attending Grambling State University, in the fall of 1976, she pledged Alpha Kappa Alpha, Sorority Incorporated; she is a *Lifetime Silver Soror.* Being a member of the sorority has afforded her the opportunity to connect with other members around the world. After graduating from Grambling, she is a kept her membership active and for the past 37 years, she has been a member of the Delta Delta Omega chapter in East St. Louis, Illinois where she has participated in various community service projects.

- Jo Ann Speer Martin

Jo Ann went into the United States Air Force in 1978 and retired as a Lieutenant Colonel in 1998. During that time she married her beloved husband, Garnel Martin, in 1986. For six years she and her husband commuted to see each other sometimes once a week and sometimes once a quarter. "Marty" as she calls him, was living in O'Fallon, already retired from the Air Force, and finishing his second career at Boeing Aircraft Company. Jo Ann was stationed/serving in Oklahoma, Indiana, and Germany while they commuted. God was with them on every trip they made back and forth to see each other. They have been married 27 years. Although Jo Ann did not give birth or raise any children, she loves Garnel's three children as if they were her own.

Jo Ann loved public speaking so she became a public speaker after she retired and traveled the country speaking for various organizations on a myriad of topics. Travelling became tiring and she decided to become a substitute teacher at Lilly Freeman Elementary School in East St Louis. After four years she took a job at First Baptist Church in O'Fallon, Illinois as the music department secretary as well as the graphic designer for church bulletins and Sunday presentations. A short time later, she became a customer service front desk person at a local YMCA where she worked for three years. While she was working, Jo Ann went back to school and became a realtor and has been a licensed realtor for the past 13 years.

Jo Ann Martin is also a member of Top Ladies of Distinction, Inc., and is Senior Vice Commander of Veterans of Foreign Wars Post 11064. She holds lifetime memberships with the Grambling State University Alumni, the NAACP, and Blacks In Government.

www.ingramcontent.com/pod-product-compliance
Lightning Source LLC
La Vergne TN
LVHW021525080426
835509LV00018B/2658